How to Get Thinner
Once and for All

How to Get Thinner Once and for All

by

Morton B. Glenn, M.D.

PRESIDENT OF THE
AMERICAN COLLEGE OF NUTRITION

E. P. DUTTON & CO., INC.

New York

DEDICATED TO THE MEMORY OF MY TEACHER,

Dr. Norman H. Jolliffe, 1901–1961

Acknowledgments

My work has brought me in contact with physicians, nutritionists, dieticians, biochemists, and others in the field of nutrition, as well as thousands of patients. I wish to acknowledge the good fortune I have had in being associated with so many people from whom I have learned so much.

I am especially indebted to the physicians and nutritionists with whom I have worked in the Bureau of Nutrition of the New York City Department of Health: for their cooperation and knowledge, for their confidence in me as well as their willingness to argue a point to its logical conclusion. The list of these people is a long one, but among them I would like to mention Miss Catherine Cowell, Supervising Nutritionist of my Morrisania Nutrition Clinic, and Mrs. Ruth Larson, Nutritionist of my Kips Bay Obesity Clinic, together with Dr. Adele Kwaszewska who has assisted me in both clinics. And special recognition goes to Dr. George Christakis, Medical Director of the Bureau of Nutrition, and to the Bureau's former director, the late Dr. Norman Jolliffe, who gave me not only knowledge, but the opportunity and encouragement to carry his work a step further. To this group I add my thanks to my secretary, Mrs. Helen Dolce, for her highly valued assistance.

Equally, I wish to acknowledge the prodding and the insistence, the encouragement, forbearance, and patience, as well as the constant devil's advocacy of my wife. Her part was well above and beyond the call of duty.

MORTON B. GLENN, M.D.

New York, New York.

Contents

10   *Contents*

Part I

Part I

Chapter 1

Your Last Diet

All of you have heard about crash diets, high protein diets, fat-free diets, egg diets, liquid-formula diets, diets requiring wonder foods or drugs, and those built around special exercises. Far too often the crash dieter finds that the scales show a rise the moment the regime ends, and so begins the seesaw existence of loss and gain that is so discouraging and demoralizing.

What, then, makes the PFI system different? It not only enables you to lose pounds but to keep them off—by teaching you *how to eat.*

My PFI diet is designed to meet the needs and the actuality of modern-day life—to make it possible for you to eat sensibly not only at home, where dieting is your responsibility, but also in social or occupational situations that present food traps. You won't have to give up your diet because you are going to a party, or out on a date, or because you are taking your biggest client to lunch. You can have sandwiches for lunch; a cocktail before dinner and wine with it; you may even have ice cream for dessert!

Your diet will not be restricted to special foods and fad gimmicks—and you will not have to rely on pills. You will not even have to count the calories—because I have already done the counting for you. You can eat as well as those slim friends you envy—once you learn about food.

These diets can be enjoyed by the gourmet, and observed as readily by the young secretary who saves her "good" meals for when she is out on dates in order to use her money for a new dress and the ever-constant stocking replacements.

There is no magic to the basic method. My PFI system is a rigid dietary approach—a group of diets designed to meet your individual needs. Each is based on a specific Portion-Frequency-Item control that has been shown to be amazingly successful and surprisingly practical. The diets define precisely what you may have, how often you may have it, and how much of it you may have. They are a unification of proven concepts well-known to the nutrition profession but rarely presented as a practical method of weight control. By this diet system, physicians and nutritionists can predict and effect weight losses to the *tenth of a pound.*

I shall devote most of this book to telling you what to do, how to do it, and when to do it. I will address you as if you were in my office and I were speaking to you personally. Many of my patients dread facing me because they feel I am never satisfied with their performance and they are fearful that I will discharge them. They accuse me of demanding results rather than asking for them. But in spite of this, these patients come back, lose weight, learn to keep their weight off, and then recommend that their friends eat their way.

And so I will be as direct and blunt with you: I will start off by asking if you are adult enough to meet a challenge. Before you answer, let me warn you that this book cannot do for you what you are unwilling to do for yourself. I can show you how to take weight off permanently, as thousands of others have done, but I personally do not take one ounce from you! Your success will require more than a desire to be thinner—it will demand your willingness to follow instructions.

I will tell you some specific stories about real people* with

---

* The stories are all based on actual people and events. In order to avoid any identification, I have combined situations into composites, with fictitious names, ages, and occupations. Any similarity with one of my patients is absolute coincidence; any similarity with readers personally unknown to me is *not* unintended.

real problems whom I have treated in hospitals, at my Obesity and Nutrition Clinics of the New York City Department of Health, as well as in my private office. I will include experiences gained when I was a Medical Consultant to the United Nations, as well as when teaching at two medical colleges.

It will also answer the questions most often asked of me by lecture audiences. I will discuss not only my theories, but the ideas of my colleagues: physicians, nutritionists, dieticians, educators, and home economists—so many of whom have spent a lifetime in nutrition; and also the knowledge of non-nutritionists who work with overweight people: psychiatrists, psychologists, and social workers. I shall not deal with fancy: everything in this book is based on scientific fact or observation.*

I have learned that though overweight people have many things in common, no two patients are exactly the same. And so I will try to cover the exceptions to the rules as well as the fine details of weight control. But I will not waste your time with the obvious.

Let's face it: you do not need anyone to tell you that cake is fattening, or that you should not eat whipped cream. But you probably do need to be told how many unwanted pounds beef and lamb can contribute—and how many fine substitutes there are. Those answers I am here to provide.

But before I go any further, I want to suggest that if you are more than 10 per cent overweight, you consult your physician about dieting. Furthermore, I must rule out some readers on medical grounds.

1) There are individuals to whom eating and overweight have such important psychological implications that dieting and weight loss might prove harmful. A large medical book has been written on this subject alone.† Fortunately, there are few people in this category.

---

* For those individuals in the medical profession who want more technical information, I suggest the chapter on obesity I wrote with Norman H. Jolliffe in *Clinical Nutrition*, 2nd ed., edited by Norman H. Jolliffe (New York: Harper, 1962).

† *The Importance of Overweight* by Hilda Bruch (New York: Norton, 1957).

2) People with diseases should let their physicians decide whether the diets outlined here are suitable.

3) Those who have food allergies should consult a doctor before embarking on these diets, for though the diets may erase symptoms caused by overconsumption, the PFI plan was not designed to cure allergies.

4) Children should not follow these diets: they were designed for adults only.

5) Pregnant or nursing women will need to have these diets modified as to amount of milk.

6) The elderly individual should not diet without his physician's advice, even though these diets have been used without major problems by an older group. Nevertheless, the older person must be willing to lose weight at a slower rate than the younger person and to pay particular attention to the avoidance of constipation. Moderate weight loss usually makes the older person look younger; extreme weight loss may do the reverse.

Unless you have a medical reason for not dieting, this book is intended for you: whether you are trying to diet for the first or the fiftieth time; whether you are long overweight or never had a weight problem until you gave up smoking; and even if you are the person who finds it easy to lose weight but all too easy to put it back.

But my book is not for the dreamer who goes to bed at night hoping to wake up thin. I can't give you the diet that lets you eat everything, the sure-cure pill that melts the fat away—the Aladdin's lamp of weight reduction.

It seems to me that every month there are magazines containing diets—*easy* ones. Yet obviously no one has discovered the perfect, easy diet for everyone; after all, the magazines keep printing new articles on new ways to lose weight.

Dieting is hard work. Following the PFI diets is no exception, but they *do* succeed. Nevertheless, it is very easy for you to prove that dieting doesn't work—and only you can prove that the PFI diet does as much for you as it has for others. There are no short cuts, and if you skip pages, you will probably shortchange yourself. If you are reading this book for dinner conversation only, try the newspaper—it is more appropriate. I am writing only for those who really mean business, who want to lose weight, who want to lose weight *now*, who want to keep it off—*once and for all*. For those to whom being thin is worth working for—hard. In our obesity clinics we discharge all patients who don't follow the diet; we mean business! If you are to lose weight, you *must* mean business. Make the diet your number one occupation—not a hobby that you engage in only when you are in the mood.

If I were giving this talk to a lecture audience, somebody would be bursting at the seams wanting to say "All this is well and good, *but* I don't have will power." So, I will now discuss just this, but don't be disappointed if I emphasize words other than will power.

What kind of effort does the PFI method of weight loss entail? Planning, deciding, care, and active doing. It is no assembly-line operation: the result should be an excellent "hand-crafted product." To achieve it, *motivation* is required—and by motivation I do not mean the fairyland wish to be thinner but *a willingness to learn a new way of eating*.

Can anyone learn a new way of eating? Recently, I attended an international nutrition meeting at which I reported on changing eating habits in a group of more than a hundred persons over the age of 60. If they can learn, so can you! But this new way of eating must also be the right way. The diet must do the following:

1) Provide you with the proper nutrition to maintain health and appearance.
2) Allow you to lose weight consistently.
3) Give you the type of training and food education that will be the basis for permanent weight-and-appetite control.

The biggest problem with weight reduction is the inability of most individuals to *maintain* their new lower weight. How many overweight persons live on the seesaw—up again, down again, up again? Even in the well-motivated patient, I have rarely observed satisfactory weight maintenance without the appropriate food education. And so, food education is essential.

But in addition to motivation and food education there is a third absolute requirement. Call it what you wish—self-discipline, self-denial, character—it's essential. Without it, lack of permanent success is practically guaranteed. I have purposely avoided the term will power, because today it seems to be reserved exclusively for the smoker or dieter. And yet it represents self-discipline—the kind we expect from all adults. The ability to practice self-denial is one of the chief distinguishing marks between the adult and the child. In which world is the individual who snatches the cookie as soon as his wife's back is turned?

Yes, dieting is tough. It takes courage and resolve. And yet many of my successful patients have said, "You know, it wasn't as tough as you said it would be."

All I really wanted them to know was that this type of dieting needs an "I mean business" attitude! It is perhaps why my patients every now and then have reported to me, "I would like to see my friend go on this diet, but it is too soon. He isn't ready for it yet." I do not know if you are ready for it, but you be the judge.

Chapter 2

What Makes People Overweight?

I am sure you know that overweight is a result of excessive eating, or of eating more food than the body uses for energy. But did you know that more than 90 per cent of overweight people are fast eaters? That the majority are stand-up eaters— people who do more eating while standing than when sitting? Or that most overweight people are such plate-cleaners that when they are through eating, their dishes look prewashed?

Let me illustrate with the story of a patient of mine, Mary J.

When I took Mary J.'s history, one fact seemed to stand out: her impatience with her eating companions. She could not understand why her sister dawdled so much over a sandwich at lunch; Mary was on her dessert before her sister finished half the sandwich. At dinner, Mary was done long before her husband and often would nibble on bread until he "caught up."

One of Mary J.'s habits while waiting for her husband to finish was to use the bread to wipe up all the gravy on her plate. After all, she had been taught as a child to clean her plate, and by the time she grew up, plate-cleaning was an obsession.

As I have said, the vast majority of overweight persons are fast eaters. They are usually done before everyone else; they take large bites; and they often act as if they know there will be no tomorrow—and they can't think of anything better to do on their last day than eat!

If you wish to lose weight, you must *start eating slowly.* It is not easy, but with a little practice it will get easier. You see, by eating rapidly you don't give the normal body processes that stop hunger enough time to come into play; hence the desire for "seconds," or to nibble while you are waiting for someone else to finish. Slow down! Your food will seem to go further. The amount of food on your PFI diet should satisfy your hunger, but you have to give your stomach a chance to send a message to your brain to tell it that the food is there. A patient of mine said that her best system was always to eat more slowly than anyone else at the table.

As for plate-cleaning, the rule is obvious: if there is more than you need on your plate, *do not eat it!* Leave that last half bite. There is no harm in forgetting some of the things you learned as a child. And if you get guilt feelings about the starving people in Asia, remember that your eating the extra food will not help them anyway. Try to take only the amount you should, but don't be afraid to leave some over.

But why, you may well ask, do I deal with matters like rapid eating before answering the complaint of many individuals: "You can't do anything for obesity—it's all psychological." So let's go into that aspect of the problem.

Just what does "it's all psychological" really mean? Psychological is an adjective defined as "pertaining to psychology," which is the science of the nature, functions, and phenomena of the human mind. Psychologically, we are of course concerned with the whys and wherefores of the overeating process and/or the emotional reactions to being overweight. After all, emotions (and their control) are an important part of *all* our lives. And eating and body weight are closely related to emotions. Eating can be a tranquilizer or a stimulant, a source of satisfaction or of failure, a source of reward or a sign of guilt, a source of protection or a symptom of vulnerability, a source of desirability or a result of rejection. It can serve many people in many ways—and it does. The list of psychological functions that are related to eating and body weight is as long as any list in a psychiatrist's dictionary. I shall discuss only those which I feel were important factors to patients I have treated.

For as I said earlier, I do not treat those who are so psychologically dependent on overweight that they need psychiatric, not dietary, help to solve their problems.

TENSION. I am personally convinced that the largest single psychological factor affecting eating and body weight is *tension*. All of our days have tensions of varying degree and duration. Sometimes a tension is fleeting, such as "Will we catch the bus?" though the problem might be severe if missing the bus meant missing an important job interview. The intensity of other emotions can be found in the answers to questions such as "Will I get caught?" "Will I get the promotion?" "Will my child survive the operation?" Some of us are a mass of tangled tensions, each tension superimposed on another, thanks to a lack of answers. Some of us have isolated but piercing tensions. Psychiatrists have always associated depression with loss of appetite, but depression is not the same as tension. Tension and frustration may result in depression, but may also result in agitation.

The vast majority of individuals have some type of eating response to tension. In my opinion, the majority of thin individuals respond to tension by a loss of appetite, the degree of loss often a measure of the degree of tension. Theirs might not be a tension of the type that will result in frustration, but perhaps the tension of a time deadline: the job becomes more important than eating. The overweight individual on the other hand finds some degree of tranquilization from eating. He gets into an argument with his wife, is upset and soon finds himself looking in the refrigerator, while the argument is still in progress. Or there is the woman who is so furious at some gossip she has just learned a friend was telling about her that she begins to eat the piece of candy her son left on the kitchen counter. Or the man who is so annoyed with the way his bridge partner is playing a hand that he heads directly to the buffet table for a piece of pastry. Or the young woman who wishes that the attractive man whom she just met will phone her, and who waits nearer the cookie jar than the telephone. Examples of this are countless.

What can be done if one eats because of tension? The answer is simple: Stop! No, I am not kidding. I am completely serious. I know how you feel: "If I could stop, I wouldn't be reading this!" But you can stop. Many psychiatrists tell alcoholics that they will be treated *only* if they stop drinking—and they do! Firstly, the person must accept the fact that he is eating because he is trying to sedate these tensions. Secondly, he must realize that all the eating will do is act as a temporary narcotic. It covers up the problem, makes it easier to take. He has to be convinced he doesn't need this protection. Most of us are built of better material than we think. How many times when I was working as an intern in the Emergency Room at Bellevue Hospital did I see a mother rush in with a severely bleeding child in her arms! She might well be a woman who under ordinary circumstances faints at the sight of blood or screams when she sees a mouse. With the life of her child at stake, though, there was no fear, no panic, no thought of self, but instead a quick-thinking, fast-moving, giant of a human being doing what had to be done. All of us have that capacity. Surely the capacities that have made the human race survive in the face of often fantastic odds are applicable to some of our smaller problems. And so the "tension eater" must learn to put his tensions in perspective, learn to handle the cause of tensions, recognize that eating doesn't eliminate the reason for the tension nor provide the solution. He must meet his problems with maturity, not narcotize them with food. If he is completely incapable of doing this—and there are few people in this category—then the source of these inabilities probably requires a more formal type of psychological assistance. This is not a Pollyanna approach, but an approach of seeing and facing the real challenges of living. It is not easy—but it can be done.

PROTECTION. Some individuals use overweight as a protective wall. They isolate themselves on an "island of fat." Some of these are people who have trouble meeting others: they actually fear meeting strangers at parties or other gatherings. Or they are frightened of the responsibilities that go with any type of relationship between two people. It is not that they do not want to know new people, make new friends, have meaningful relationships, but they have an *inner fear of these relationships,* their responsibilities and challenges. An almost sure way to protect oneself against these potential challenges (and often they include the challenge of marriage!) is to be unattractive, and what easier way is there to be unattractive than to be fat? Of course, this is mostly an unconscious type of thinking. It is not common, but not rare either. Understanding requires much insight, and sometimes professional help.

One of my patients was a man in his late thirties who was a consultant engineer. During the day he had little contact with women; he spent his evenings alone. His colleagues urged him to lose weight, and so he started a weight reduction program with me. His evening boredom presented a problem, and I encouraged him to join a discussion group that met once or twice a week at the YMCA-YWCA. I felt that this would offer him a constructive and enjoyable way to spend some of his evenings, and give him an opportunity to meet some women. He took my advice, and enjoyed the discussion groups and the new friends he made. He was self-conscious about his weight at first, but this passed quickly. Then something unexpected happened. He began to cheat on his diet. Close analysis of his daily dietary records revealed his cheating was confined to those days that he was to attend the discussion group. This observation was confirmed by the fact that on one occasion when his work prevented him from going to the group he followed his diet perfectly. It became apparent that he was "hiding behind his fat"; really making himself unattractive to the opposite sex; avoiding the relationships he thought he wanted! After much discussion, despite his attempts at evasion, we gained enough insight to see the true mechanisms. He sought psychiatric aid and with very few visits to the psychiatrist is now a "new man." He is losing weight and making a much better adjustment to the world around him.

Again I say that though there are many, many psychological problems that could be discussed here, most overweight people do not require psychiatric treatment to handle their problems.

All of us handle psychological situations daily: dealing with a spouse, a child, an unwilling buyer, a difficult employer, a harsh landlord, a boy friend, a grouchy delivery man, etc. Most of us are quite capable of dealing with these situations. Most of us are equally quite capable of dealing with the psychological problems involved in weight reduction.

SMOKING. It is difficult to talk about the relationship between psychology and weight reduction without considering smoking, or rather giving up smoking, and what that does to weight gain. There has been so much publicity about smoking that few smokers haven't read that theirs is an "oral drive." An oral drive is an inner force to put something in the mouth, whether it be food, gum, cigarettes, fingernails, or a pencil. All people, thin or fat, smokers or non-smokers, have such a drive to some degree—some much stronger than others. But just because a man is overweight or is a heavy smoker doesn't necessarily mean that he has a strong oral drive.

Smoking for most people is a habit that is perpetuated and reinforced by its continuation. This habit ultimately involves more than just the inhalation of smoke. It involves the lighting and the holding of the cigarette—a hand occupation as well as a mouth occupation. Cigarettes also have a tranquilizing effect on tensions. Inasmuch as the giving up of cigarettes doesn't mean that there is a giving up of tensions, most smokers tend to use the hand and oral approach to continue the sedation originally afforded by cigarettes. Eating is an almost reflex way of attaining a similar type of gratification. Because additional food means extra weight, a large number of individuals who stop smoking start gaining unless they follow a preventive program.

If you plan to stop smoking and are worried about what that will do to your weight, I would suggest the following: concentrate on the between-meal time. Since the extra eating comes at a time when you would ordinarily be smoking, mealtime is rarely a problem, except possibly the end of a meal. So, take an extra cup of coffee at the end of the meal (without milk, cream, or sugar), but not an extra dessert. In fact, do not stay at the table any longer than you must. And between meals, if you find the need to eat something almost impossible to overcome, try carrots or celery, more black coffee, or water—yes, just plain water. Your desire to eat these extras will gradually diminish as time goes on. Also, occupy your hands. It helps. Some people have suggested the use of an empty cigarette holder. This may help for a while, but sooner or later you will have to give that up also.

If you are overweight and wish to give up smoking and go on a diet at the same time, *don't!* The simultaneous approach *can* be achieved, but rarely. Give up the cigarettes first, and meanwhile follow the preventive program described above to avoid any further weight gain. When you have definitely stopped smoking—give yourself three to six months to prove it—then start the full dietary program outlined in this book.

If you have already given up smoking, and have thereby gained weight, then simply follow the plan of weight reduction outlined throughout this book.

Most people who give up smoking find that there is a gradual increase in eating, and a gradual increase in weight (unless the above preventive program is started). After a while, their weight levels off. If you did not have a preventive program, start your diet here. Do not delay!

And do not be deluded into thinking that if you are overweight, smoking will control your appetite. It won't!

CHAPTER 3

A Visit to My Office

To give you a better idea of what goes on with other over-weight people, let me tell you how I deal with a new patient.

The visitor sees the usual desk and chairs with a small double bench and end table. There is the scale of course, which probably looks a little larger to my patients than it really is (it is made specially for me but is standard size), and pasted on it is the rather ugly, but important, annual seal of accuracy of the Bureau of Weights and Measures. There are the usual medical books as well as the medical magazines that seem to come in faster than one can read them; some water colors done by my wife; and a collection of wax food models. These wax models are quite realistic: it looks as though I have various parts of a meal (steak, ice cream, etc.) strewn about my desk. I use these food models to demonstrate portion sizes to my patients.

Now for that first interview. My secretary showed in a new patient, Mrs. Pierce. Mrs. Pierce was just a few years past forty; her face seemed quite relaxed, but she was toying nervously with the handle of her pocketbook. Almost before I had a chance to say anything, she quickly blurted, "My husband will be in to see you later this week. We both want to diet together." And then she added, "I have to lose weight right away." The suddenness of this type of statement is not surprising. Who doesn't want to lose weight right away?

27

I told her that I looked forward to meeting her husband, and pointed out that it is often helpful for a husband and wife to diet at the same time. It makes life a little easier for each of them (unless of course this turns out to be a competitive couple, in which case we can be in for a difficult time). But I also asked her what the rush was. She explained that her daughter was going to get married in four months: "And I'm *not* going to look fat at the wedding."

Mrs. Pierce wanted to lose weight fast. I told her I could give her a diet which would result in her losing almost two pounds per week. "What?" she almost screamed. "I have about twenty pounds to lose; I can't wait that long. I don't have the time to do it slowly!"

I explained that she would be losing weight at the rate of about 100 pounds per year; how could that be considered slow? I also explained that even if I put her on a true starvation diet of water alone—not even one calorie's worth of food —she probably would not lose more than 4½ pounds per week after the first 7 to 10 days of dieting.

"Besides," I reminded her, "you will have more problems with eating than you anticipate: showers, between-shopping lunches with your daughter, tea with your son-in-law's mother, all the extra dinners and get-togethers for relatives, celebration parties. . . . With the work in store for you—no matter how pleasurable—you certainly cannot afford to endanger your health by bad dieting. Furthermore, if you do undertake a crash diet, do you know how you might look at the end of it? Massive weight losses often give you badly wrinkled skin. I can put you on a diet that you will not only enjoy—though you will still have to work hard at it—but that will also teach you the habits that will enable you to maintain your new weight. After all, you'll still be seeing the in-laws after the wedding. As far as timing is concerned, let me say that even though you can probably afford to lose 25 instead of 20 pounds, you can do this in about 14 to 15 weeks. Since the wedding is 4 months off, we may even have a few weeks to spare and to meet the last dress fitting."

After this explanation, I started taking a history to learn

as much as I could about Mrs. Pierce. What was her weight as a child, as a teen-ager, at her marriage? How much did she gain during her pregnancies? What did she weigh five years ago, two years ago, one year ago, now? Then a family history: What was the weight situation of her parents, her brothers and sisters, her children? Did she ever suffer from any diseases that might interfere with her dieting? How did she feel now? Overly tired? Short of breath? Did she have indigestion? (These are the typical overweight person's complaints. Incidentally, I once had a patient who denied indigestion, but who six weeks after starting his diet announced, "You know, Doctor, I haven't taken any antacid pills for weeks now!")

From here I went on to her social history. Where was she born? How much schooling did she have? How did she usually spend her day? Had she a job? What kind? And then to her eating patterns, both past and present.

Was she a frequent dieter? Was she on the seesaw of weight gain and weight loss? Was she a fussy eater? Did a "good eating time" consist of a lot of bread and butter, or did it mean fancy eating with special sauces and foreign food? Was she a plate-cleaner, and if so was she taught this as a child? Had there been food deprivation in childhood? Was she a fast or slow eater? Also, did she use salt excessively? Did she prefer spicy foods? Was she one of those individuals who salted before tasting?

Did she ever hoard food? Keep it in a drawer or closet? Or was she a secret eater—eating only when her husband wasn't looking? Did her parents yell at her for being fat when she was young, or were they constantly trying to make her eat? And now—was anyone nagging her about her weight? And then I went on to ask whether her appetite increased with tension, whether she had any food allergies, any foods she refused to eat no matter what the circumstances, any religious restrictions on her eating. Finally, we covered her actual intake. We had now truly bared her "eating soul." When the frequent or constant dieter discusses openly all these phases of her eating life, the frank discussion (almost a confession) allows us to start with a completely clean slate. Under this type of questioning, I have found my patients to be completely truthful with but one exception: when I ask a woman what size dress she wears. If it's a fight between a size 18 and 20, I am always told that a 16 is getting too small! How do I know this? After a diet is over, I usually ask my patient what size dress she is wearing. She announces with much pride her new size, and when I comment how nice it is that she is no longer a tight 16, I get a smiling statement about the fight between the 18 and 20.

I measured Mrs. Pierce's height and weighed her. When she saw what she weighed, she was shocked. Her comment was "The air must be heavier here than in my home."

I laughed and told her I hadn't heard that excuse before.

She was indignant. "I'm not kidding. After all, I see the seal of the Bureau of Weights and Measures on your scale, so your scale must be correct. But I'm certain my scale is correct too. It's a doctor's scale, you know, and my scale was three pounds less this morning. It must be the air!"

I was a little embarrassed for having laughed, but explained the probabilities. Most people who have scales at home weigh themselves on arising, after going to the toilet, and before dressing. Since this was after breakfast, the difference between the two scales really represented the weight of her clothing and breakfast. She now understood everything—and I hope no one else suggests there might be a problem with heavy air.

Mrs. Pierce got the question I ask of all patients on their first visit: "Why are you overweight?" Today, wisely, almost all answer: "I eat too much" or words of similar kind.

Formerly the most common answer was "sluggish metabolism" or "my glands." Since some individuals still feel that metabolism or glands are the cause of their overweight, I wish to discuss this point.

Metabolism refers to the body processes or cell chemical changes by which food is converted into living tissue and by which living tissue is then broken down to more simple compounds. The building up and the breaking down of tissue are all accompanied by an exchange of energy. When we measure metabolism, we usually measure the energy exchange. The unit of energy that we use for measurements is the calorie. In very technical terms, a calorie is the quantity of heat required to raise the temperature of 1000 grams (1 kilogram) of water 1 degree Centigrade. A given amount of food will contain a certain number of calories, or in other words, a certain amount of energy is available for body use from this foodstuff. These calories are "burned" in the body to form tissues and usable chemicals. Some foods, such as fats, have a larger number of calories (more energy) per unit of weight than do proteins, sugars, and starches. As the chemicals and tissues are broken down, there is also an energy exchange, which is again measurable as calories. Throughout every moment of our lives we are constantly absorbing energy from foods and at the same time spending it as we break down various compounds and tissues. Living is therefore a constant building up and breaking down of cellular compounds. The *rate* of this building up and breaking down is the metabolic rate. Since every little motion of our lives affects this rate, we measure it best in a resting, or basal, condition. That is why we call the test a basal metabolism test. Our answers can be shown in calories used per minute or per hour, but for practical purposes, we give the answer in the percentage above or below average. Since it is difficult to get a precise answer, we then consider any result from 10 per cent above to 10 per cent below as normal.

To return to the term sluggish metabolism, its actual meaning is that a person not only has trouble spending energy but also has difficulty in building tissue, and what overweight person ever complains of this? Besides, heavy people need more energy to carry their weight about (just as a car with an extra load in the trunk uses extra gas). So if anything, most overweight people burn more energy than do thin people.

Even individuals who have diseases associated with very low basal metabolic rates are usually not obese, no matter which gland is the seat of the disorder. Besides, this book is not for those with proven severe glandular diseases. It is for those who would lose weight by eating less. Leave the glandular care to your physician. Leave the getting thinner to your diet.

Back to Mrs. Pierce. I told her that it was necessary to verify some physical facts. I gave her a brief physical examination and took some blood for laboratory tests. I then said that I would explain her diet to her after I received the results of her blood tests. (We can now make some metabolism determinations by the use of blood iodine tests, and though, as I have stressed, it is not at all common for my patients to have unusual metabolic problems, I like to make sure.) We arranged that at her next appointment, I would go over the details of the diet with both her and her husband, in order to save them time: though their requirements would probably be different, the basic information would not.

Meanwhile, I had an appointment with Mr. Pierce, who turned out to be jolly and fat. He'd been fat for ten years and though he was used to it, he was tired of all the old jokes about his weight. Moreover, he was truly concerned— more so than he would ever had admitted to his wife. Now, since his daughter was getting married, and his wife was really going to diet, he felt that this would be a good opportunity for him too. I took a history similar to the one I described for Mrs. Pierce. We discussed the major things— what he ate, when he ate them. Also little things: Did he "chisel" cookies from his secretary? What did he really mean by a "healthy" portion? Did he take a quick bite or two or three or four in the kitchen while waiting for his wife to serve dinner? Was he embarrassed to order cottage cheese at a business luncheon when his client ordered steak? When his wife nagged about his weight, did he sometimes get angry enough to take another bite for spite?

THE MEAT QUESTION. Mr. Pierce answered me frankly, but he made it clear he really could not understand why he was overweight. After all, he stuck to steak and chops most of the time and didn't order potatoes very much: so why should he be fat? Besides, he didn't even eat desserts very often. Of course, after I found out about all of his eating habits, I could see many flaws in his diet pattern. But without going into that for now, let's direct ourselves to his specific question about "steak and chops and very little potatoes."

Believe it or not, the *highest calorie foods per portion*—and by portion I am referring to that size usually served and eaten in the U.S.—are beef, pork, and lamb! Yes, beef, pork, and lamb. Did you ever take cold steak wrapped in aluminum foil out of the refrigerator? Did you notice those little gleaming yellowish-white spots that covered both the meat and the foil? They're fat! And the fat did not come from the foil! It's there when the steak is hot, but you can't see it simply because fat melts when hot. Since a great part of Mr. Pierce's diet was beef, you can see that his was a high fat diet—even though he thought it was solely a high protein diet. Protein is good for you—in fact, essential—and meat is an excellent source of protein. But you know the story: two aspirins can cure a headache, while a bottle of aspirins may kill you. And so, just because beef, pork, and lamb are nutritious, they are good for the overweight person only if taken in the right amount.

What then *is* the right amount?

I told Mr. Pierce I would put him on a PFI diet that had a total of 1500 calories a day. He looked astonished and said, "I can't lose weight on 1000 calories, so how can I lose it on 1500?"

When I explained that a one-pound boneless prime porterhouse (which he had previously stated he could consume in no time flat) might contain 1500 calories, he began to listen with new intensity. The light had struck! Maybe, he started to realize, his 1000-calorie diet was nearer 10,000! But then he added quickly, "I stick to lean meat: choice or prime only."

Just what is the meaning of *choice* and *prime* meats? The chief characteristic of these top grades is their fat content. *A high fat content!* Utility meats are of much lower fat content. Thus the better the grade, the more fat that is present! (By the way, what I say for beef includes pork and lamb as well—though there is usually more fat in pork than in either beef or lamb.)

Mr. Pierce had used the term "healthy" portion. Just what is a healthy portion? A large one? Why equate *large* with *healthy*? What is so healthy about a pound of meat loaded with fat? I am not suggesting that one eat low grades of meat, but I am stressing that the best grades of these meats are not without a high fat content. To put it simply, choice and prime indicates fine, not lean.

By now you may wonder what kind of diet I gave to Mr. Pierce. Let me say quickly it was not without meat. Every meal in the PFI diet includes an animal protein. By that I mean protein derived from animals rather than from plants (which are called vegetable protein).

How can I criticize fatty foods and still allow beef and lamb? By seeing to it that my patients pay attention to portions and frequency.

Both Mr. and Mrs. Pierce returned a few days later for their diet explanations. At this time I calculated the amount of weight each should lose weekly, and drew personal graphs for each of them. I explained their diets and answered all their questions.

I saw them weekly in the office. They both were diligent and were doing well. I advised Mrs. Pierce that if she were ever tempted to go off her diet, even for the briefest moment, she should think of what size gown she would wear at the wedding. One day she told me that she had a better way of keeping to her regimen: "Billy, that's my daughter's fiancé Billy's mother is as thin as a rail. I am darned if she will ever have the opportunity to say that her son's mother-in-law was fat!"

She progressed beautifully. About ten weeks after she started the diet, she gave a big Thanksgiving dinner. The week after Thanksgiving she reported, "You know, this dinner was a new experience for me. I've been on the diet for only ten weeks, and I can no longer eat those large portions. I am embarrassed to say it, but for the first time I had the impression that my relatives were making pigs of themselves.

My husband couldn't keep up with them either. And when all the other men decided to take a walk around the block after dinner, I decided that at next year's dinner I am going to use smaller plates. Maybe then the family will take smaller portions."

She never returned after that visit, but soon after the wedding I received a letter from Mr. Pierce. A newspaper announcement was enclosed and next to it were a few words penned in a quick hand: "And the bride's mother said to tell you she wore a size 10!"

The letter included the following note: "And now when we look at a steak dinner, we say to each other: 'Can we afford a fattening dinner?'"

CHAPTER 4

What Should You Weigh?

One of the questions I ask my patients on their very first visit is what they would like to weigh. But I am always careful to bury this question among many others and to change the subject as soon as I have recorded their answers. I especially avoid any discussion of the issue, for, in the course of the diet, most of my successful patients change their goals. Over two-thirds of my patients, when within 5 to 10 pounds of their original objective, have told me they want to lose even more. Why is this? Many patients who have been on the weight seesaw for a long time think *only* in terms of the easiest achievable goal. Granted, they are out to lose weight—but seldom enough, for their ideal weight level seems as remote to them as the possibility of a million-dollar inheritance. And who likes to aim at unrealistic goals?

I, in turn, don't want to impose a severe goal, whether real or apparent, because to the patient the time necessary to achieve it will loom as "forever." So I take the patient's estimate as a temporary goal and concentrate on how to achieve it.

In the beginning, therefore, our only goal is going to be a weekly one. And incidentally, there is no point in wishing you good luck. DIETING AND LUCK ARE UNRELATED.

Part II

Part II

CHAPTER 1

On Your Mark, Get Set, Go!

Well, let's get started—now! Put down that piece of fruit you are eating. Now means this very second, and your diet shall continue every second of every minute and every minute of every hour, weekday or weekend, holiday or workday—until you get to the right weight. There can be no tomorrow in dieting. You know that yourself. How many times have you promised yourself, "I'll start my diet tomorrow"—and what happened?

As I said right at the beginning, your diet is designed for you whether you are eating at home or in somebody else's home; it works equally well in your kitchen, your friend's kitchen, or your relative's kitchen. And the dining room, bedroom, living room, or foyer won't affect it either. The diet can follow you to restaurants, luncheonettes, delicatessens, or night clubs. It works whether you are eating on the job or while going to school. It goes with you to weddings and funerals, parties and religious festivals—and on vacation. There is no vacation from health and there is no vacation from a diet! And it allows for no excuses. So put all your excuses in a safety deposit box and throw away the key!

But right at the start, let me tell you there is one word that we never use: try. All too many of you are reading this book because you have tried, tried, and tried again. So forget the word *try* and substitute *do!* Anyone who has ever been on a diet knows the difference between the two.

Remember, the only time you get into trouble on a diet is when you cheat a second time. And the only way you can avoid cheating a second time is by not cheating a first time. A simple concept—but very true. It is much more difficult to stop after the first peanut than before!

There are two parts to the PFI diets: the first covers the basic rules for everyone who is overweight; the second is made up of specific instructions to meet individual needs.

Your diet will be nutritionally sound as well as adjustable to your social, business, and home needs. The diets for women have sufficient latitude to allow the sixty-year-old widow, the young mother, the single career girl, or the middle-aged woman to follow them. There is an equal amount of latitude in the diets for men to provide both for the advertising executive who does most of his business over a big lunch and for the manual worker who takes a lunch box. The diets, then, are constructed with a rigid outer framework but with adjustable interiors.

Since you will be learning new eating habits, some of them will be strange to you. Parts of the diet requirements may even seem to give you *too much* to eat—but you must eat it. Parts will seem just right to you. And I know very well that there will be others which you feel do not allow you enough to eat. You will also find that some of the food items permitted are both familiar and delightful, while others will not appeal to you at the start. At times you will feel quite full; other times only partially satisfied; but rarely if ever dissatisfied. And if you do become hungry occasionally, remember your motivation!

Every food in the world is regarded from three points of view:

1) Is it allowed or not? This is known as *item control.*
2) If allowed, how often can it be had? Daily? And if so, how many times a day? Or is it allowed only a certain number of times in a week? Throughout the diet explanations, the *frequency control* will be detailed. Unless

I state otherwise, any item allowed in a meal can be had at each meal of that type.

3) When allowed, how large is each individual serving? Just what is the *portion control*?

You must learn item control, frequency control, and portion control for every foodstuff! One is as important as the others. Too much of the "right" food is just as bad as any of the wrong foods!

You must also accept the fact that every detail counts. Nothing is unimportant. The success of your diet depends on details. For example, sampling is not allowed—no matter how small the taste. Your diet may permit you half a grapefruit, but that doesn't include the maraschino cherry. Did you know that the amount of syrup which comes with the cherry is equivalent to a lump of sugar? So remember: throw away the cherry unless the diet specifies its inclusion.

Now let's go through the list of foods by item and frequency standards; the portions are determined by your individual diet, but the general rules of preparation remain the same and so are included at the end of each category. (Detailed instructions for purchasing, cooking, and serving are given later in the book.)

MEATS, FISH, SHELLFISH, AND POULTRY

ITEM CONTROL

FORBIDDEN (because of excessive fat content)
Pork. All types: fresh, canned, or mixtures with other substances. This includes bacon, ham, and most frankfurters. (Unless frankfurters are labeled "all beef," they usually are made of pork.)
Beef sweetbreads
Corned beef
Duck
Fish packed in oil (except salmon)
Goose
Pastrami

ALLOWED

All other forms of meat, fish, shellfish, and poultry, but subject to the following frequency control.

FREQUENCY CONTROL

Do not exceed the frequency of serving or the size of the portion listed in your specific diet. If I were asked to pick the most important instruction in the entire book, this would be it.

A. LIMITED TO 3 LUNCH PORTIONS AND 4 DINNER PORTIONS PER WEEK:

> Beef
> Beef tongue
> Bismarck herring (smoked)
> Bologna
> Fresh salmon
> Lamb
> Liverwurst
> Turkey (dark meat)

B. MORE FREQUENTLY ALLOWED. The following animal proteins are preferable to beef and lamb, and may be had whenever your diet calls for meat, fish, shellfish, or poultry. But they too may be eaten *only* in those amounts called for in your diet. Portion control is just as important with these foods as with beef and lamb. Incidentally, these other animal proteins are plentiful, and most are quite inexpensive, though a few are expensive. At any rate, these include:

> Beef heart
> Chicken
> Fish
> Kidneys (including pork)
> Liver
> Lungs
> Roe

Sardines (in tomato or mustard sauce only!)
Shellfish
Turkey (white meat)
Veal

Remember, every time you replace beef and lamb with either fish, shellfish or poultry, *the better off* you are. To remind yourself of this hourly is barely enough.

If at any time, no "flesh food" is available for dinner, then as an emergency you may substitute two eggs or cottage cheese in an amount equal to 1½ times the portion of meat you are allowed (for example, for 4 ounces of meat use 6 ounces of cottage cheese) or hard cheese in an amount equal to half the meat portion you are allowed (for 4 ounces of meat, use 2 ounces of hard cheese).

C. UNDETERMINED ALLOWANCE: TIRED LEOPARDS. I include so odd an item because somebody always asks me the calorie count of an unusual food. If the food item is really a rarity, frankly I cannot tell you whether it is allowed or not. I am concerned in this book with the common needs—not the rare ones.

But if you are interested, I will give you a list of some of the game foods. The real reason for this list is not that I want to favor the hunter but that the unusual items may make you refer to the list more than once. It may also get you to reread these paragraphs! The following are some game foods:

Consider as poultry-fish equivalents:

Armadillo
Goat
Guinea hen
Muskrat
Pheasant
Quail
Venison
Wild rabbit
Whale

Consider as beef equivalents:

Alligator
Opossum
Raccoon
Squab
Wild duck

PREPARATION

Since you are concerned with the fat content of meat, you would defeat your diet if you added any fat in the cooking. Therefore, you may use no fat, oil, lard, butter, or margarine whatsoever in the cooking. Believe it or not, foods can be broiled *and be tasty* without the addition of any of the above. If you are worried that the meat will dry out too much, baste it with heated consommé, lemon juice, or tomato juice.

The ideal method of cooking is to broil over an open rack (the kind found in most ordinary ovens). This allows the fat to drip off. Granted, you will have to scrub your broiler, but it is better to let the steel wool rather than your stomach lining deal with the extra fat! Though you can bake, roast, or boil, you may not pan-broil: then the food really fries in its own fat!

What do you mean you cannot cook lobster without butter? You can boil it: many gourmets like boiled lobster best. And if you omit the drawn butter, you will discover the true taste of lobster. Steamed clams? Certainly, but only if you plan to dip them in the clam broth—not in butter. Incidentally, have you ever tried vealburgers? They are excellent and less fatty than beefburgers.

VEGETABLES

Vegetables are considered in two main categories: raw and cooked. The cooked ones are to be taken only at mealtime in accordance with your diet plan. The raw ones are for salads or sandwiches (I told you sandwiches would be allowed!) and as a between-meal snack.

RAW VEGETABLES

SALADS. They are always allowed on all diets at both lunch and dinner. If you are so inclined, you may have salad at breakfast also, but I must admit I have had only one patient who ever did this. But salads are subject to the following rules:

They must consist of nothing but vegetables. No fruit (no avocados, no nuts) except for tomatoes—and even then, only one tomato per day. If you wish, you may make a jellied salad by using unsweetened gelatin with or without some tomato juice.

You may eat any type of *raw* vegetable in *any* amount (except for tomatoes, as explained above). A green salad may be as large as you want it. Of course, if you consume the entire contents of a vegetable store in one sitting, you are working against the diet—and yourself. Again I say, anyone can prove a diet doesn't succeed: it takes you to prove it *does!*

While salads are not required—eat them or not as you like—I recommend them strongly as a good source of vitamins, minerals, and bulk. They help to complete and round out your meals. They are a great filler. Besides, they add food to your diet!

DRESSING. Your leeway with salads does not extend to salad dressings. The only dressings allowed are:

Dietetic dressing
Lemon
Spices
Tomato juice
Vinegar

Or any combination of these. But be particularly careful about the dietetic dressings: there are right and wrong ones. Just because a label says "low-calorie" doesn't mean it is suitable for your purposes. *Read the* BACK *label.* It must say the dressing contains *less than* 3 calories per teaspoon or less than 7 calories per tablespoon. So read that label carefully.

Of course, if you are going to put a gallon of even a permitted dietetic dressing on every salad, you won't be helping your cause any. Use a reasonable amount.

And teach yourself this: no oil; no mayonnaise. Don't bother looking for a dietetic mayonnaise. Though I don't know *all* the brands sold throughout the country, I do not know of any mayonnaise that meets the "less than 3 calories per teaspoon" requirement. By the way, coleslaw almost always contains mayonnaise, so rule out coleslaw unless you are absolutely certain it is made with vinegar only.

Again I point out that salads are good. Eat them—but with no exceptions to the rules!

SANDWICHES. If you dislike salads, why not take your raw vegetables in sandwich form? You may add lettuce and tomato to any sandwich your diet allows.

For BETWEEN-MEAL SNACKS, raw vegetables are perfect: they may be eaten at any time, in any amount, *at any time* of the day or night. That is, if you wish and when you wish—without restriction.

COOKED VEGETABLES

Cooked vegetables, too, supply vitamins and minerals, and add the bulk needed for good bowel function.

I realize that many of you do not think you like vegetables, but perhaps you haven't given them a fair chance. Have you ever, as a guest at someone's home, been served a vegetable you had never tasted but assumed was horrible—and then discovered it wasn't so bad after all?

Don't be afraid to be adventurous. At worst, you may confirm your dislike of a particular vegetable; at best, you may discover a whole new food world.

ITEM CONTROL

FORBIDDEN

Beans (except string beans or wax beans, which are allowed)
Chick peas
Corn
Dried peas or lentils or dried soybeans
Noodles
Potatoes
Rice
Spaghetti and macaroni
Yams

ALLOWED

All other vegetables, including canned and frozen ones —unless the package says "sugar added."

Measuring portions. Though the number of cooked vegetables you may have varies in accordance with your diet plan, the definition of a portion is always the same:

1 portion = ½ cup of cooked vegetable.

In other words, measure *after*, not *before*, cooking.

If for any medical reason, you must use puréed, baby, junior, or salt-free vegetables, you will need to know that 3½ ounces of the bottled or canned vegetable is the equivalent of the ½-cup serving; the weight is given on the label.

FREQUENCY CONTROL

You may never have more than ½ cup of the SAME *vegetable within a 48-hour period.* This is essential—a rule which must be observed both at lunch and at dinner.

Whenever I mention this to a patient in the office, I get a quizzical look in response, and so I had better explain carefully. If your diet restricts you to ½ cup of a cooked vegetable, you have only to choose which one you want. But if your diet allows you 1 cup (2 portions) of cooked vegetables at a meal, you are to have ½ cup each of two different vegetables—*not* one full cup of one vegetable. Similarly, when your diet gives you a choice of 1 or 2 portions, it does not mean that the 2 portions may be of the same vegetable. And once you have a portion of cooked vegetable, you may not repeat it for the next 48 hours.

The purpose of this restriction is to encourage a greater variety—to allow you a wider choice—without in any way upsetting the caloric balance of your diet. If you are wondering where you will find enough vegetables to fill this requirement, let me tell you that one nutrition book listing vegetables in alphabetical order has 37 just for the letters A, B, and C!

PREPARATION

Though any method of cooking vegetables is allowed *except frying*, the best way is to steam them in a pressure cooker, after you put a small amount of liquid in the pot. Use the vitamin-rich liquid from the vegetables either as a sauce for them or as stock for basting meats.

Whatever your method of preparation, remember one thing: *you may never use—either during or after cooking—any fat, oil, butter, margarine, or lard.* Do not be shocked. Vegetables can be made to taste fine without any of these. Salt is allowed. Spices are allowed. You may even use some of the milk from your daily milk quota. Besides, the main lesson most people have to learn—for the sake of taste and nutrition—is not to overcook. If you are careful about this, you won't need to rely on fats to make vegetables a gourmet's delight.

FRUITS*

ITEM CONTROL

FORBIDDEN
Cherries
Grapes
Watermelon

---

* Tomatoes are discussed under Salads.

Amazed? My patients always are when they hear this. So before I name the other forbidden fruits, let me tell you why these three are on the list.

I know that watermelon has only 28 calories per half cup. But do you know any watermelon-liker who will be satisfied with half a cup of watermelon balls? And did you know that the usual size wedge—⅛ of an average watermelon (i.e., ¼ of a half melon)—contains 500 calories? And if you really have a watermelon appetite and eat ¼ of a melon, as some people do, you are getting 1000 calories. If you are on a 1000-calorie diet, you have used up the whole day's allowance. Of course, if you order watermelon in a restaurant which serves really small portions, you may get 250 calories. But 250 calories happens to be 3½ times the count allowed for *each* fruit portion.

We really forbid watermelon because of the practical impossibility of controlling portion size. For the same reason we forbid grapes and cherries; they are usually consumed by the bagful. A pound of cherries is about 250 calories; a pound of grapes even more. So no watermelon, grapes, or cherries, unless they are part of a fruit cup and the total portion is not more than ½ cup.

The other fruits on the forbidden list are:

> Avocados
> Canned fruit, *unless dietetic or water-packed*
> Dried fruits such as apricots, dates, figs, prunes, and raisins
> Frozen berries, or any frozen fruit (unless the package specifically says "no sugar added": most of them are packed in sugar before freezing)
> Fruit jelly, jam, preserves, or marmalade (*including the dietetic ones*)
> Fruit sauces or toppings
> Maraschino cherries: even one is too many
> Olives

The term dietetic is often used for canned fruits which contain a sugar substitute but no additional juice or syrup. The term water-packed is usually used when there is neither additional juice nor sugar substitutes. The reason you cannot have sugar-packed fruit is that even if you washed it thoroughly in hot water to dissolve the sugar, you could not take out all of the extra sugar in the juice and syrup: some of it has become part of the fruit.

ALLOWED

All other fruits.

FREQUENCY CONTROL

The number of servings daily are in accordance with your diet plan. Vary your fruits, but if you must choose a favorite, do choose cantaloupe. It is the most filling and the lowest in calories.

PORTION CONTROL

All fruits *must* be medium-sized. You need not purchase the miniature fruit, but you must certainly avoid the large "Bon Voyage" size. Do not fool yourself. As I have said repeatedly, it is your job to prove that the diet works.

Consider a whole medium-sized fruit as one portion, then, and note the following rules for other sizes:

1) Large-sized fruit (banana, grapefruit, mango, papaya, persimmon, and pomegranate): ½ equals one portion.
2) Smaller-sized fruit (apricots, fresh dates, fresh figs, nectarines, plums): 2 or 3 constitute a portion.
3) Very small-sized fruit (fruit cup and fresh berries) as well as cooked fruit (such as applesauce and rhubarb): ½ cup makes 1 portion. Remember, these food items must never be sweetened with sugar.
4) Melons: Except for cantaloupe, a melon portion consists of 1/6 of an average melon (a section about 2 inches wide at the largest point). A cantaloupe portion is ½ of a small (5 inches in diameter) melon. But remember, no watermelon of any size.

FRUIT JUICES

ITEM CONTROL

FORBIDDEN
Guava juice, pomegranate juice, and prune juice

ALLOWED
In place of one fruit portion, you may substitute the following fruit *juices* (but *not* fruit drinks) in ½-cup (4-ounce) portions:

Apple	Loganberry
Apricot juice and nectar	Orange
Blackberry	Orange and pineapple
Blueberry	Papaya
Currant	Peach nectar
Grape	Pineapple
Grapefruit	Raspberry
Grapefruit and orange	Tangerine

These juices, however, are allowed only if they are *not sweetened with sugar* (check the labels). There is no objection to *artificially* sweetened juices in 4-ounce amounts.

FREQUENCY CONTROL

Be careful not to substitute fruit juice for whole fruits all the time. The fiber in the whole fruit provides bulk that is necessary for good bowel function.

PORTION CONTROL

As stated before, one fruit serving is equal to 4 ounces of fruit juice with the following exceptions:

Cranberry, lemon, lime, and tomato juice may be used in full cup (8-ounce) portions, if not sweetened with sugar.

NUTS

No nuts or nut products are allowed—not even one! Have you ever tried *not* to eat a second peanut after eating the first?

Did you know that 4 medium Brazil nuts have more calories than a glass of skim milk? No, no nuts allowed. And remember, coconut is a nut, and peanut butter is made from nuts.

BREADS AND OTHER BAKED GOODS

FORBIDDEN

The following breads and other baked goods are not allowed for one of the following reasons: they are too high in calories; too difficult to measure or control as to portion sizes; or they lack proper nutritional qualities for this diet.

Bagels	French bread
Biscuits	Italian bread
Bread sticks	Muffins
Buns	Nut breads
Cakes of any description	Pastry
Cookies	Pies
Corn bread	Pizzas
Crackers	Popovers
Danish	Raisin bread
Doughnuts	Rolls (hard or soft)
Fortune cookies	Salt sticks

Some types of bread substitutes are allowed occasionally—but not regularly.

In place of:

1 "regular" slice of bread:	*1 "thin" slice of bread:*
½ matzoth square, or	⅓ matzoth square, or
3 Rye Krisp, or	2 Rye Krisp, or
3 Melba toast	2 Melba toast

As to toasting—it matters not. Toast or do not, as you prefer. About the only effect of toasting is a small loss of thiamine (Vitamin B-1).

ALLOWED

Enriched cracked wheat
Enriched white
Light rye (see discussion)

Protein
Whole wheat

For your diet we deal with "basic" breads. Enriched means vitamins added, not calories. It is expected that all bread eaten at home shall be *thin-sliced*. It is only when you are out for lunch that it is permissible to eat a whole slice of *regular* bread. Most breads that are labeled "diet bread" contain fewer calories per slice than the average only because the bread is thinly sliced! Sliced bread is usually (though not always) packaged in 1-pound units of 16 slices—so that each slice weighs approximately 1 ounce. Diet breads usually have about 21 or 22 slices to the pound, roughly ⅔ of an ounce to the slice. You might feel silly counting bread slices, but once you do, you will have no problem thereafter. Be particularly careful of rye bread. It may look thin-sliced, but be so wide or so compact and free of air that it may weigh 1 ounce or more per slice. If in doubt, do not eat the rye bread. Choose from the other permitted breads instead.

Incidentally, did you know that some pumpernickels derive their rich brown color not from any magic substance native to the rich brown earth, but from the addition of molasses or caramel? In other words, by the addition of a form of sugar: unnecessary extra calories!

SPECIAL WARNING

Please reread the list of forbidden baked goods. I specified *no cake of any description*, and I am sorry to say that includes the following:

1) Birthday cake. Even your own. If you wish, you may feel sorry for yourself, but do *not* eat it. Remember, you are the one who wants to lose weight!

2) Your daughter's very first self-baked cake. Perhaps you can suggest that she bring it intact to Grandma and Grandpa—they will relish the visit. If you must try it, though, keep yours one tiny taste with much smacking of the lips! And for her second cake employ more tact and *no* tasting!

To sum up the rules just covered:

MEAT, POULTRY, FISH AND SHELLFISH

Use lean cuts only; trim away all visible fat.

Use fish, shellfish, and poultry in place of meat as often as possible.

Do not have more than 4 beef or lamb dinner servings per week.

Do not have more than 3 beef or lamb lunch servings per week.

Broil, boil, bake, or roast only. Preferably broil over open rack.

NO ham, pork, bacon, sausage; NO duck or goose; NO beef sweetbreads; NO corned beef, pastrami, or luncheon meats.

NO thick gravies, cheese or cream sauces, catsup, or chili sauce.

VEGETABLES

Salads: Any uncooked vegetable may be used in any amount, but no avocados, and never more than one tomato.

NO dressing except lemon and/or vinegar or *some* dietetic dressings (but no dietetic mayonnaise).

Cooked vegetables: Boil, steam, or bake only. Use NO butter, fat, oleomargarine, or oil; NO cream or cheese sauces.

NO potatoes, yams, spaghetti, macaroni, or noodles.

NO lima beans, rice, or corn.

1 portion = ½ cup; *NEVER* have more than ½ cup of the same cooked vegetable in a 48-hour period.

FRUITS

1 portion = 1 medium-sized fruit; 2 halves of canned (dietetic or water-packed) fruit; or ½ cup of small-sized fruit; ½ cup of cooked fruit;

Or ½ small cantaloupe or wedge (1/6) of other melons (except watermelon), or ½ banana.

NO watermelon, grapes, or cherries; frozen berries or any other frozen fruit packed in sugar; nuts or dried fruits (dates, figs, prunes, raisins, apricots).

BREAD AND OTHER BAKED GOODS
NO rolls, muffins, cake, pie, pastry, cookies, or crackers.

WHAT TO TAKE WHEN:

Hungry	*Thirsty*
raw carrots or celery	water or club soda
tea or coffee (plain)	tea or coffee (plain)
bouillon	dietetic soda

If there are any doubts—DON'T EAT IT!
R-E-M-E-M-B-E-R: Do not let your hunger and appetite rule you!
Let your better judgment be the ruler of what you eat!

If all this sounds too difficult, close the cover and put the book down. Consider giving it to a friend, the nearest library, or use it to prop up a short leg on a table. If you cannot follow these rules, this diet is not for you!

CHAPTER 2

The Right Diet for You

Now that you have learned the basic rules, the next thing you must do is find out which PFI diet was designed for you. To do this, estimate in round numbers how much overweight you think you are. On the following pages are two sets of tables, one for women and one for men, arranged according to height (without shoes). Pick your table; check for your age bracket; then read across to find the diet letter for the amount of weight you wish to lose. Remember your diet letter. Immediately under the letter, you will find a number which indicates approximately how many pounds you will lose each week by following this diet.

As you will see, the charts start with a 20-pound overweight category. If you are *less than 10 pounds* overweight, choose for your diet the preceding letter. For example, if the 20-pound overweight diet for your height and age is Diet D, you should select Diet C in order to lose less than 10 pounds. Otherwise, all the rules apply to you that apply to the heavier patient. You must spend the weeks necessary to learn new eating habits, so read the book as carefully as if you were much more overweight.

If you have *less than 5 pounds to lose*, concentrate particularly on avoiding beef and lamb. But again follow through on all the basic principles discussed in the book.

On the other hand, if you spend ¾ of your working day

in a manual labor job, then choose the diet letter *following* the one indicated by the chart. (Example: if the chart says you should choose Diet D, but you do manual labor, then choose Diet E.)

After you have lost 20 pounds, go back to your chart and check the diet letter for the next lower category: this will indicate whether your diet and weekly weight loss must now change.

To sum up how to use these charts assume that you are a woman, 5′3″ tall, 45 years old, and 40 pounds overweight.

1) Turn to p. 67 for your diet selection chart.
2) Read down to the 40–49 age group.
3) Read across to the 40-pound overweight column where you will find Diet C. This is your diet letter.
4) On this diet you should lose 2 pounds per week.
5) After you have lost 20 pounds, go back to the chart and check the diet letter for those 20 pounds overweight.
6) It shows that you should change to Diet B, with a weight loss of 2¼ pounds per week.

You might be interested to know that I use the following diets for the majority of patients I see:

Women—Diet C
Men—Diet D
Male manual workers—Diet E

DIET SELECTION CHART
(and expected weekly weight loss)

WOMEN <u>4</u> Ft. <u>9</u> In.

	If you are overweight by:						
	20 lbs.	40 lbs.	60 lbs.	80 lbs.	100 lbs.	150 lbs.	200 lbs.
Age 18–19:							
Select diet	C	C	C	C	C	C	D
Expected wkly. weight loss	2	2	2½	2½	2½	3	2¾
Age 20–29:							
Select diet	B	C	C	C	C	C	C
Expected wkly. weight loss	2	1¾	1¾	2	2¼	2½	3
Age 30–39:							
Select diet	B	B	C	C	C	C	C
Expected wkly. weight loss	1¾	1¾	1¾	1¾	2	2½	2¾
Age 40–49:							
Select diet	B	B	C	C	C	C	C
Expected wkly. weight loss	1¾	1¾	1½	1¾	2	2¼	2¾
Age 50–59:							
Select diet	B	B	C	C	C	C	D
Expected wkly. weight loss	1½	1¾	1½	1¾	1¾	2¼	2
Age 60–69:							
Select diet	B	B	B	C	C	D	D
Expected wkly. weight loss	1	1¼	1½	1¼	1½	1¼	1½
Age 70–79:							
Select diet	A	B	B	B	C	–	–
Expected wkly. weight loss	1¼	1	1¼	1½	1¼	–	–

DIET SELECTION CHART

(*and expected weekly weight loss*)

WOMEN 4 Ft. 10 In.

If you are overweight by:

	20 lbs.	40 lbs.	60 lbs.	80 lbs.	100 lbs.	150 lbs.	200 lbs.
Age 18–19:							
Select diet	C	C	C	C	C	C	D
Expected wkly. weight loss	2	2¼	2¼	2½	2½	3	2¾
Age 20–29:							
Select diet	B	C	C	C	C	C	C
Expected wkly. weight loss	2	1¾	2	2	2½	2¾	3
Age 30–39:							
Select diet	B	B	C	C	C	C	C
Expected wkly. weight loss	1¾	2	1¾	2	2	2½	3
Age 40–49:							
Select diet	B	B	C	C	C	C	C
Expected wkly. weight loss	1¾	2	1¾	1¾	2	2¼	2¾
Age 50–59:							
Select diet	B	B	C	C	C	C	D
Expected wkly. weight loss	1¾	1¾	1½	1¾	2	2¼	2
Age 60–69:							
Select diet	B	B	B	C	C	D	D
Expected wkly. weight loss	1¼	1¼	1½	1¼	1½	1¼	1½
Age 70–79:							
Select diet	A	B	B	B	C	–	–
Expected wkly. weight loss	1¼	1	1¼	1½	1¼	–	–

DIET SELECTION CHART

(and expected weekly weight loss)

WOMEN   <u>4</u> Ft. <u>11</u> In.

If you are overweight by:

	20 lbs.	40 lbs.	60 lbs.	80 lbs.	100 lbs.	150 lbs.	200 lbs.
Age 18–19:							
Select diet	C	C	C	C	C	C	D
Expected wkly. weight loss	2	2¼	2¼	2½	2¾	3	3
Age 20–29:							
Select diet	C	C	C	C	C	C	C
Expected wkly. weight loss	1¾	1¾	2	2¼	2¼	2¾	3
Age 30–39:							
Select diet	B	C	C	C	C	C	C
Expected wkly. weight loss	2	1¾	1¾	2	2¼	2½	3
Age 40–49:							
Select diet	B	C	C	C	C	C	C
Expected wkly. weight loss	1¾	1½	1¾	2	2	2½	2¾
Age 50–59:							
Select diet	B	B	C	C	C	C	D
Expected wkly. weight loss	1¾	1¾	1½	1¾	2	2¼	2¼
Age 60–69:							
Select diet	B	B	B	C	C	D	D
Expected wkly. weight loss	1¼	1½	1½	1¼	1½	1¼	1¾
Age 70–79:							
Select diet	B	B	B	C	C	–	–
Expected wkly. weight loss	1	1¼	1¼	1	1¼	–	–

DIET SELECTION CHART

(*and expected weekly weight loss*)

WOMEN <u>5</u> Ft. <u>0</u> In.

If you are overweight by:

	20 lbs.	40 lbs.	60 lbs.	80 lbs.	100 lbs.	150 lbs.	200 lbs.
Age 18–19:							
Select diet	C	C	C	C	C	C	D
Expected wkly. weight loss	2¼	2¼	2½	2½	2¾	3¼	3
Age 20–29:							
Select diet	C	C	C	C	C	C	C
Expected wkly. weight loss	1¾	2	2	2¼	2¼	2¾	3¼
Age 30–39:							
Select diet	B	C	C	C	C	C	C
Expected wkly. weight loss	2	1¾	2	2	2¼	2½	3
Age 40–49:							
Select diet	B	C	C	C	C	C	C
Expected wkly. weight loss	1¾	1½	1¾	2	2	2½	3
Age 50–59:							
Select diet	B	C	C	C	C	C	D
Expected wkly. weight loss	1¾	1½	1¾	1¾	2	2½	2¼
Age 60–69:							
Select diet	B	B	C	C	C	D	D
Expected wkly. weight loss	1¼	1½	1¼	1¼	1½	1½	1¾
Age 70–79:							
Select diet	B	B	B	C	C	–	–
Expected wkly. weight loss	1	1¼	1½	1¼	1¼	–	–

DIET SELECTION CHART

(and expected weekly weight loss)

WOMEN <u>5</u> Ft. <u>1</u> In.

If you are overweight by:

	20 lbs.	40 lbs.	60 lbs.	80 lbs.	100 lbs.	150 lbs.	200 lbs.
Age 18–19:							
Select diet	C	C	C	C	C	C	D
Expected wkly. weight loss	2¼	2½	2½	2¾	3	3¼	3
Age 20–29:							
Select diet	C	C	C	C	C	C	C
Expected wkly. weight loss	1¾	2	2	2¼	2½	2¾	3¼
Age 30–39:							
Select diet	B	C	C	C	C	C	C
Expected wkly. weight loss	2	1¾	2	2	2¼	2¾	3
Age 40–49:							
Select diet	B	C	C	C	C	C	C
Expected wkly. weight loss	1¾	1¾	1¾	2	2¼	2½	3
Age 50–59:							
Select diet	B	C	C	C	C	C	D
Expected wkly. weight loss	1¾	1½	1¾	2	2	2½	2¼
Age 60–69:							
Select diet	B	B	C	C	C	D	D
Expected wkly. weight loss	1¼	1½	1¼	1½	1½	1½	1¾
Age 70–79:							
Select diet	B	B	B	C	C	—	—
Expected wkly. weight loss	1	1¼	1½	1¼	1¼	—	—

DIET SELECTION CHART

(and expected weekly weight loss)

WOMEN <u>5</u> Ft. <u>2</u> In.

	If you are overweight by:						
	20 lbs.	40 lbs.	60 lbs.	80 lbs.	100 lbs.	150 lbs.	200 lbs.
Age 18–19:							
Select diet	C	C	C	C	C	C	D
Expected wkly. weight loss	2¼	2½	2¾	2¾	3¼	3¾	3½
Age 20–29:							
Select diet	C	C	C	C	C	C	C
Expected wkly. weight loss	1¾	2	2¼	2¼	2½	3	3¼
Age 30–39:							
Select diet	B	C	C	C	C	C	C
Expected wkly. weight loss	2	2	2	2¼	2¼	2¾	3¼
Age 40–49:							
Select diet	B	C	C	C	C	C	C
Expected wkly. weight loss	2	1¾	2	2¼	2¼	2½	3
Age 50–59:							
Select diet	B	C	C	C	C	C	D
Expected wkly. weight loss	2	1¾	2	2	2¼	2½	2½
Age 60–69:							
Select diet	B	B	C	C	C	D	D
Expected wkly. weight loss	1½	1½	1¼	1½	1¾	1½	2
Age 70–79:							
Select diet	B	B	B	C	C	–	–
Expected wkly. weight loss	1¼	1¼	1½	1¼	1½	–	–

DIET SELECTION CHART
(*and expected weekly weight loss*)

WOMEN <u>5</u> Ft. <u>3</u> In.

	If you are overweight by:						
	20 lbs.	40 lbs.	60 lbs.	80 lbs.	100 lbs.	150 lbs.	200 lbs.
Age 18–19:							
Select diet	C	C	C	C	C	C	D
Expected wkly. weight loss	2½	2½	2¾	3	3	3½	3¼
Age 20–29:							
Select diet	C	C	C	C	C	C	D
Expected wkly. weight loss	2	2	2¼	2½	2½	3	2¾
Age 30–39:							
Select diet	B	C	C	C	C	C	C
Expected wkly. weight loss	2¼	2	2¼	2¼	2½	2¾	3¼
Age 40–49:							
Select diet	B	C	C	C	C	C	C
Expected wkly. weight loss	2¼	2	2	2¼	2½	2¾	3¼
Age 50–59:							
Select diet	B	C	C	C	C	C	D
Expected wkly. weight loss	2	1¾	2	2	2¼	2¾	2½
Age 60–69:							
Select diet	B	B	C	C	C	D	D
Expected wkly. weight loss	1½	1¾	1½	1½	1¾	1½	2
Age 70–79:							
Select diet	B	B	B	C	C	—	—
Expected wkly. weight loss	1¼	1½	1½	1¼	1½	—	—

DIET SELECTION CHART

(and expected weekly weight loss)

WOMEN <u>5</u> Ft. <u>4</u> In.

If you are overweight by:

	20 lbs.	40 lbs.	60 lbs.	80 lbs.	100 lbs.	150 lbs.	200 lbs.
Age 18–19:							
Select diet	C	C	C	C	C	C	D
Expected wkly. weight loss	2½	2¾	3	3	3¼	3½	3½
Age 20–29:							
Select diet	C	C	C	C	C	C	C
Expected wkly. weight loss	2	2¼	2½	2½	2¾	3	3½
Age 30–39:							
Select diet	C	C	C	C	C	C	C
Expected wkly. weight loss	2	2	2¼	2½	2½	3	3¼
Age 40–49:							
Select diet	C	C	C	C	C	C	C
Expected wkly. weight loss	1¾	2	2¼	2¼	2½	3	3¼
Age 50–59:							
Select diet	C	C	C	C	C	C	D
Expected wkly. weight loss	1¾	2	2	2¼	2½	2¾	2½
Age 60–69:							
Select diet	C	C	C	C	C	D	D
Expected wkly. weight loss	1¼	1½	1½	1¾	1¾	1¾	2
Age 70–79:							
Select diet	B	C	C	C	C	—	—
Expected wkly. weight loss	1¼	1	1¼	1½	1½	—	—

DIET SELECTION CHART

(and expected weekly weight loss)

WOMEN 5 Ft. 5 In.

If you are overweight by:

	20 lbs.	40 lbs.	60 lbs.	80 lbs.	100 lbs.	150 lbs.	200 lbs.
Age 18–19:							
Select diet	C	C	C	C	C	C	D
Expected wkly. weight loss	2¾	2¾	3	3¼	3¼	3¾	3½
Age 20–29:							
Select diet	C	C	C	C	C	C	D
Expected wkly. weight loss	2¼	2¼	2½	2¾	2¾	3¼	3
Age 30–39:							
Select diet	C	C	C	C	C	C	C
Expected wkly. weight loss	2	2¼	2¼	2½	2¾	3	3½
Age 40–49:							
Select diet	C	C	C	C	C	C	C
Expected wkly. weight loss	2	2	2¼	2½	2½	3	3¼
Age 50–59:							
Select diet	C	C	C	C	C	C	D
Expected wkly. weight loss	1¾	2	2¼	2¼	2½	3	2¾
Age 60–69:							
Select diet	C	C	C	C	C	D	D
Expected wkly. weight loss	1¼	1½	1¾	1¾	2	1¾	2¼
Age 70–79:							
Select diet	C	C	C	C	C	–	–
Expected wkly. weight loss	1	1¼	1¼	1½	1¾	–	–

DIET SELECTION CHART

(and expected weekly weight loss)

WOMEN <u>5</u> Ft. <u>6</u> In.

If you are overweight by:

	20 lbs.	40 lbs.	60 lbs.	80 lbs.	100 lbs.	150 lbs.	200 lbs.
Age 18–19:							
Select diet	C	C	C	C	C	D	D
Expected wkly. weight loss	2¾	3	3	3¼	3½	3¼	3½
Age 20–29:							
Select diet	C	C	C	C	C	C	D
Expected wkly. weight loss	2¼	2½	2½	2¾	3	3¼	3
Age 30–39:							
Select diet	C	C	C	C	C	C	D
Expected wkly. weight loss	2¼	2¼	2½	2½	2¾	3¼	3
Age 40–49:							
Select diet	C	C	C	C	C	C	D
Expected wkly. weight loss	2	2¼	2¼	2½	2¾	3	2¾
Age 50–59:							
Select diet	C	C	C	C	C	C	D
Expected wkly. weight loss	2	2	2¼	2½	2½	3	2¾
Age 60–69:							
Select diet	C	C	C	C	D	D	E
Expected wkly. weight loss	1½	1½	1¾	2	1½	1¾	1¾
Age 70–79:							
Select diet	C	C	C	C	C	–	–
Expected wkly. weight loss	1¼	1¼	1½	1½	1¾	–	–

DIET SELECTION CHART

(and expected weekly weight loss)

WOMEN 5 Ft. 7 In.

If you are overweight by:

	20 lbs.	40 lbs.	60 lbs.	80 lbs.	100 lbs.	150 lbs.	200 lbs.
Age 18–19:							
Select diet	C	C	C	C	C	D	D
Expected wkly. weight loss	3	3	3¼	3½	3½	3¼	3¾
Age 20–29:							
Select diet	C	C	C	C	C	C	D
Expected wkly. weight loss	2¼	2½	2¾	2¾	3	3½	3¼
Age 30–39:							
Select diet	C	C	C	C	C	C	D
Expected wkly. weight loss	2¼	2½	2½	2¾	3	3¼	3
Age 40–49:							
Select diet	C	C	C	C	C	C	D
Expected wkly. weight loss	2	2¼	2½	2½	2¾	3	3
Age 50–59:							
Select diet	C	C	C	C	C	D	D
Expected wkly. weight loss	2	2¼	2½	2½	2¾	2½	3
Age 60–69:							
Select diet	C	C	C	C	D	D	E
Expected wkly. weight loss	1½	1¾	1¾	2	1½	2	1¾
Age 70–79:							
Select diet	C	C	C	C	C	–	–
Expected wkly. weight loss	1¼	1½	1½	1¾	1¾	–	–

DIET SELECTION CHART
(*and expected weekly weight loss*)

WOMEN <u>5</u> Ft. <u>8</u> In.

	If you are overweight by:						
	20 lbs.	40 lbs.	60 lbs.	80 lbs.	100 lbs.	150 lbs.	200 lbs.
Age 18–19:							
Select diet	C	C	C	C	C	D	D
Expected wkly. weight loss	3	3¼	3¼	3½	3¾	3½	3¾
Age 20–29:							
Select diet	C	C	C	C	C	C	D
Expected wkly. weight loss	2½	2½	2¾	3	3	3½	3¼
Age 30–39:							
Select diet	C	C	C	C	C	C	D
Expected wkly. weight loss	2¼	2½	2¾	2¾	3	3½	3¼
Age 40–49:							
Select diet	C	C	C	C	C	C	D
Expected wkly. weight loss	2¼	2¼	2½	2¾	2¾	3¼	3
Age 50–59:							
Select diet	C	C	C	C	C	C	D
Expected wkly. weight loss	2¼	2¼	2½	2¾	2¾	2½	3
Age 60–69:							
Select diet	C	C	C	D	D	D	E
Expected wkly. weight loss	1½	1¾	2	1½	1½	2	1¾
Age 70–79:							
Select diet	C	C	C	D	D	–	–
Expected wkly. weight loss	1¼	1½	1½	1¼	1¼	–	–

DIET SELECTION CHART

(and expected weekly weight loss)

WOMEN <u>5</u> Ft. <u>9</u> In.

If you are overweight by:

	20 lbs.	40 lbs.	60 lbs.	80 lbs.	100 lbs.	150 lbs.	200 lbs.
Age 18–19:							
Select diet	C	C	C	C	C	D	E
Expected wkly. weight loss	3	3¼	3½	3½	3¾	3½	3¼
Age 20–29:							
Select diet	C	C	C	C	C	C	D
Expected wkly. weight loss	2½	2¾	3	3	3¼	3½	3½
Age 30–39:							
Select diet	C	C	C	C	C	C	D
Expected wkly. weight loss	2¼	2½	2¾	3	3	3½	3¼
Age 40–49:							
Select diet	C	C	C	C	C	C	D
Expected wkly. weight loss	2¼	2½	2½	2¾	3	3¼	3
Age 50–59:							
Select diet	C	C	C	C	C	D	D
Expected wkly. weight loss	2¼	2½	2½	2¾	3	2¾	3
Age 60–69:							
Select diet	C	C	D	D	D	E	E
Expected wkly. weight loss	1¾	1¾	1½	1½	1¾	1½	2
Age 70–79:							
Select diet	C	C	C	D	D	–	–
Expected wkly. weight loss	1¼	1½	1½	1¼	1½	–	–

DIET SELECTION CHART

(*and expected weekly weight loss*)

WOMEN <u>5</u> Ft. <u>10</u> In.

If you are overweight by:

	20 lbs.	40 lbs.	60 lbs.	80 lbs.	100 lbs.	150 lbs.	200 lbs.
Age 18–19:							
Select diet	C	C	C	C	D	D	E
Expected wkly. weight loss	3¼	3½	3½	3¾	3¼	3¾	3½
Age 20–29:							
Select diet	C	C	C	C	C	C	D
Expected wkly. weight loss	2½	2¾	3	3¼	3¼	3¾	3½
Age 30–39:							
Select diet	C	C	C	C	C	C	D
Expected wkly. weight loss	2½	2¾	3	3	3¼	3½	3½
Age 40–49:							
Select diet	C	C	C	C	C	C	D
Expected wkly. weight loss	2½	2½	2¾	2¾	3	3½	3¼
Age 50–59:							
Select diet	C	C	C	C	C	D	E
Expected wkly. weight loss	2¼	2½	2¾	2¾	3	2¾	2½
Age 60–69:							
Select diet	C	C	D	D	D	E	E
Expected wkly. weight loss	1¾	2	1½	1½	1¾	1½	1¾
Age 70–79:							
Select diet	C	C	C	D	D	—	—
Expected wkly. weight loss	1½	1½	1¾	1¼	1½	—	—

DIET SELECTION CHART

(and expected weekly weight loss)

WOMEN <u>5</u> Ft. <u>11</u> In.

If you are overweight by:

	20 lbs.	40 lbs.	60 lbs.	80 lbs.	100 lbs.	150 lbs.	200 lbs.
Age 18–19:							
Select diet	C	C	C	D	D	E	E
Expected wkly. weight loss	3¼	3½	3¾	3¼	3½	3¼	3½
Age 20–29:							
Select diet	C	C	C	C	C	D	D
Expected wkly. weight loss	2¾	3	3	3¼	3½	3¼	3½
Age 30–39:							
Select diet	C	C	C	C	C	C	D
Expected wkly. weight loss	2¾	2¾	3	3¼	3¼	3¾	3½
Age 40–49:							
Select diet	C	C	C	C	C	C	D
Expected wkly. weight loss	2½	2¾	2¾	3	3	3½	3¼
Age 50–59:							
Select diet	C	C	C	C	D	D	E
Expected wkly. weight loss	2½	2½	2¾	3	2½	3	2¾
Age 60–69:							
Select diet	C	D	D	D	D	E	F
Expected wkly. weight loss	1¾	1½	1½	1¾	2	1¾	1¾
Age 70–79:							
Select diet	C	C	D	D	D	–	–
Expected wkly. weight loss	1½	1¾	1¼	1½	1½	–	–

DIET SELECTION CHART

(*and expected weekly weight loss*)

WOMEN   <u>6</u> Ft. <u>0</u> In.

If you are overweight by:

	20 lbs.	40 lbs.	60 lbs.	80 lbs.	100 lbs.	150 lbs.	200 lbs.
Age 18–19:							
Select diet	C	C	D	D	D	E	E
Expected wkly. weight loss	3½	3¾	3¼	3¼	3½	3¼	3¾
Age 20–29:							
Select diet	C	C	C	C	C	D	D
Expected wkly. weight loss	2¾	3	3¼	3¼	3½	3¼	3¾
Age 30–39:							
Select diet	C	C	C	C	C	C	D
Expected wkly. weight loss	2¾	3	3	3¼	3½	3¾	3½
Age 40–49:							
Select diet	C	C	C	C	C	D	D
Expected wkly. weight loss	2½	2¾	3	3	3¼	3	3½
Age 50–59:							
Select diet	C	C	C	D	D	D	E
Expected wkly. weight loss	2½	2¾	3	2½	2½	3	2¾
Age 60–69:							
Select diet	D	D	D	D	E	E	F
Expected wkly. weight loss	1¼	1½	1¾	1¾	1½	1¾	1¾
Age 70–79:							
Select diet	D	D	D	D	D	–	–
Expected wkly. weight loss	1	1¼	1¼	1½	1¾	–	–

DIET SELECTION CHART

(and expected weekly weight loss)

MEN <u>5</u> Ft. <u>0</u> In.

If you are overweight by:

	20 lbs.	40 lbs.	60 lbs.	80 lbs.	100 lbs.	150 lbs.	200 lbs.
Age 18–19:							
Select diet	D	D	D	D	D	D	E
Expected wkly. weight loss	2½	2½	2¾	3	3	3½	3¼
Age 20–29:							
Select diet	D	D	D	D	D	D	E
Expected wkly. weight loss	1¾	1¾	2	2¼	2¼	2¾	2½
Age 30–39:							
Select diet	C	D	D	D	D	D	D
Expected wkly. weight loss	2	1½	1½	1¾	2	2½	2¾
Age 40–49:							
Select diet	C	C	C	D	D	D	D
Expected wkly. weight loss	1¾	2	2	1¾	1¾	2¼	2½
Age 50–59:							
Select diet	C	C	C	D	D	D	D
Expected wkly. weight loss	1¾	2	2	1½	1¾	2¼	2½
Age 60–69:							
Select diet	C	C	C	C	D	D	E
Expected wkly. weight loss	1¼	1½	1¾	1¾	1½	1¾	1½
Age 70–79:							
Select diet	B	C	C	C	C	–	–
Expected wkly. weight loss	1¼	1	1¼	1½	1½	–	–

DIET SELECTION CHART

(*and expected weekly weight loss*)

MEN <u>5</u> Ft. <u>1</u> In.

	If you are overweight by:						
	20 lbs.	40 lbs.	60 lbs.	80 lbs.	100 lbs.	150 lbs.	200 lbs.
Age 18–19:							
Select diet	D	D	D	D	D	D	E
Expected wkly. weight loss	2½	2¾	2¾	3	3¼	3½	3½
Age 20–29:							
Select diet	D	D	D	D	D	D	E
Expected wkly. weight loss	1¾	2	2	2¼	2½	2¾	2½
Age 30–39:							
Select diet	D	D	D	D	D	D	D
Expected wkly. weight loss	1½	1¾	1¾	2	2	2½	3
Age 40–49:							
Select diet	C	C	D	D	D	D	D
Expected wkly. weight loss	2	2	1½	1¾	2	2¼	2¾
Age 50–59:							
Select diet	C	C	D	D	D	D	E
Expected wkly. weight loss	1¾	2	1½	1¾	1¾	2¼	2
Age 60–69:							
Select diet	C	C	C	C	D	D	E
Expected wkly. weight loss	1¼	1½	1½	1¾	1¼	1¾	1½
Age 70–79:							
Select diet	C	C	C	C	D	–	–
Expected wkly. weight loss	1	1¼	1¼	1½	1	–	–

DIET SELECTION CHART

(and expected weekly weight loss)

MEN <u>5</u> Ft. <u>2</u> In.

	If you are overweight by:						
	20 lbs.	40 lbs.	60 lbs.	80 lbs.	100 lbs.	150 lbs.	200 lbs.
Age 18–19:							
Select diet	D	D	D	D	D	D	E
Expected wkly. weight loss	2¾	2¾	3	3¼	3¼	3¾	3½
Age 20–29:							
Select diet	D	D	D	D	D	D	E
Expected wkly. weight loss	2	2	2¼	2½	2½	3	2¾
Age 30–39:							
Select diet	D	D	D	D	D	D	D
Expected wkly. weight loss	1½	1¾	2	2	2¼	2¾	3
Age 40–49:							
Select diet	D	D	D	D	D	D	D
Expected wkly. weight loss	1½	1½	1¾	1¾	2	2½	2¾
Age 50–59:							
Select diet	C	D	D	D	D	D	E
Expected wkly. weight loss	2	1½	1½	1¾	2	2¼	2¼
Age 60–69:							
Select diet	C	C	C	D	D	D	E
Expected wkly. weight loss	1¼	1½	1¾	1¼	1½	1¾	1½
Age 70–79:							
Select diet	C	C	C	C	D	–	–
Expected wkly. weight loss	1	1¼	1½	1½	1	–	–

DIET SELECTION CHART

(*and expected weekly weight loss*)

MEN 5 Ft. 3 In.

If you are overweight by:

	20 lbs.	40 lbs.	60 lbs.	80 lbs.	100 lbs.	150 lbs.	200 lbs.
Age 18–19:							
Select diet	D	D	D	D	D	E	E
Expected wkly. weight loss	2¾	3	3	3¼	3½	3¼	3¾
Age 20–29:							
Select diet	D	D	D	D	D	D	E
Expected wkly. weight loss	2	2¼	2½	2½	2¾	3	3
Age 30–39:							
Select diet	D	D	D	D	D	D	E
Expected wkly. weight loss	1¾	2	2	2¼	2¼	2¾	2½
Age 40–49:							
Select diet	D	D	D	D	D	D	D
Expected wkly. weight loss	1½	1¾	1¾	2	2	2½	3
Age 50–59:							
Select diet	C	D	D	D	D	D	E
Expected wkly. weight loss	2	1½	1¾	1¾	2	2½	2¼
Age 60–69:							
Select diet	C	C	C	D	D	D	E
Expected wkly. weight loss	1½	1½	1¾	1¼	1½	1¾	1¾
Age 70–79:							
Select diet	C	C	C	D	D	–	–
Expected wkly. weight loss	1¼	1¼	1½	1	1¼	–	–

DIET SELECTION CHART

(and expected weekly weight loss)

MEN <u>5</u> Ft. <u>4</u> In.

If you are overweight by:

	20 lbs.	40 lbs.	60 lbs.	80 lbs.	100 lbs.	150 lbs.	200 lbs.
Age 18–19:							
Select diet	D	D	D	D	D	E	E
Expected wkly. weight loss	3	3	3¼	3½	3½	3¼	3¾
Age 20–29:							
Select diet	D	D	D	D	D	D	E
Expected wkly. weight loss	2¼	2¼	2½	2¾	2¾	3¼	3
Age 30–39:							
Select diet	D	D	D	D	D	D	D
Expected wkly. weight loss	1¾	2	2¼	2¼	2½	3	3¼
Age 40–49:							
Select diet	D	D	D	D	D	D	D
Expected wkly. weight loss	1½	1¾	2	2	2¼	2½	3
Age 50–59:							
Select diet	D	D	D	D	D	D	E
Expected wkly. weight loss	1½	1¾	1¾	2	2	2½	2¼
Age 60–69:							
Select diet	C	C	D	D	D	D	E
Expected wkly. weight loss	1½	1¾	1¼	1½	1½	2	1¾
Age 70–79:							
Select diet	C	C	C	D	D	–	–
Expected wkly. weight loss	1¼	1½	1½	1	1¼	–	–

DIET SELECTION CHART

(and expected weekly weight loss)

MEN <u>5</u> Ft. <u>5</u> In.

	If you are overweight by:						
	20 lbs.	40 lbs.	60 lbs.	80 lbs.	100 lbs.	150 lbs.	200 lbs.
Age 18–19:							
Select diet	D	D	D	D	D	E	F
Expected wkly. weight loss	3	3¼	3¼	3½	3¾	3½	3½
Age 20–29:							
Select diet	D	D	D	D	D	D	E
Expected wkly. weight loss	2¼	2½	2½	2¾	3	3¼	3
Age 30–39:							
Select diet	D	D	D	D	D	D	D
Expected wkly. weight loss	2	2	2¼	2½	2½	3	3½
Age 40–49:							
Select diet	D	D	D	D	D	D	D
Expected wkly. weight loss	1¾	1¾	2	2¼	2¼	2¾	3
Age 50–59:							
Select diet	D	D	D	D	D	D	E
Expected wkly. weight loss	1½	1¾	2	2	2¼	2½	2½
Age 60–69:							
Select diet	C	D	D	D	D	E	E
Expected wkly. weight loss	1½	1¼	1¼	1¼	1¾	1½	1¾
Age 70–79:							
Select diet	C	C	C	D	D	–	–
Expected wkly. weight loss	1¼	1¼	1¾	1¼	1¼	–	–

DIET SELECTION CHART

(*and expected weekly weight loss*)

MEN <u>5</u> Ft. <u>6</u> In.

If you are overweight by:

	20 lbs.	40 lbs.	60 lbs.	80 lbs.	100 lbs.	150 lbs.	200 lbs.
Age 18–19:							
Select diet	D	D	D	D	E	E	F
Expected wkly. weight loss	3¼	3¼	3½	3¾	3¼	3½	3½
Age 20–29:							
Select diet	D	D	D	D	D	D	E
Expected wkly. weight loss	2½	2½	2¾	3	3	3½	3¼
Age 30–39:							
Select diet	D	D	D	D	D	D	D
Expected wkly. weight loss	2	2¼	2½	2½	2¾	3	3½
Age 40–49:							
Select diet	D	D	D	D	D	D	D
Expected wkly. weight loss	1¾	2	2	2¼	2½	2¾	3¼
Age 50–59:							
Select diet	D	D	D	D	D	D	E
Expected wkly. weight loss	1¾	1¾	2	2¼	2¼	2¾	2½
Age 60–69:							
Select diet	C	D	D	D	D	E	E
Expected wkly. weight loss	1¾	1¼	1½	1½	1¾	1½	2
Age 70–79:							
Select diet	C	C	C	D	D	–	–
Expected wkly. weight loss	1½	1½	1¾	1¼	1½	–	–

DIET SELECTION CHART
(*and expected weekly weight loss*)

MEN <u>5</u> Ft. <u>7</u> In.

	If you are overweight by:						
	20 lbs.	40 lbs.	60 lbs.	80 lbs.	100 lbs.	150 lbs.	200 lbs.
Age 18–19:							
Select diet	D	D	D	D	E	E	F
Expected wkly. weight loss	3¼	3½	3½	3¾	3¼	3¾	3¾
Age 20–29:							
Select diet	D	D	D	D	D	D	E
Expected wkly. weight loss	2½	2¾	2¾	3	3¼	3½	3¼
Age 30–39:							
Select diet	D	D	D	D	D	D	E
Expected wkly. weight loss	2¼	2¼	2½	2¾	2¾	3¼	3
Age 40–49:							
Select diet	D	D	D	D	D	D	D
Expected wkly. weight loss	2	2	2¼	2½	2½	3	3¼
Age 50–59:							
Select diet	D	D	D	D	D	D	E
Expected wkly. weight loss	1¾	2	2	2¼	2½	2¾	2½
Age 60–69:							
Select diet	C	D	D	D	D	E	E
Expected wkly. weight loss	1¾	1¼	1½	1¾	1¾	1½	2
Age 70–79:							
Select diet	C	C	D	D	D	–	–
Expected wkly. weight loss	1½	1½	1¼	1¼	1½	–	–

DIET SELECTION CHART

(*and expected weekly weight loss*)

MEN 5 Ft. 8 In.

	If you are overweight by:						
	20 lbs.	40 lbs.	60 lbs.	80 lbs.	100 lbs.	150 lbs.	200 lbs.
Age 18–19:							
Select diet	D	D	D	E	E	F	G
Expected wkly. weight loss	3½	3½	3¾	3¼	3½	3½	3½
Age 20–29:							
Select diet	D	D	D	D	D	D	E
Expected wkly. weight loss	2¾	2¾	3	3	3¼	3¾	3½
Age 30–39:							
Select diet	D	D	D	D	D	D	E
Expected wkly. weight loss	2¼	2½	2¾	2¾	3	3¼	3¼
Age 40–49:							
Select diet	D	D	D	D	D	D	D
Expected wkly. weight loss	2	2¼	2¼	2½	2¾	3	3½
Age 50–59:							
Select diet	D	D	D	D	D	E	E
Expected wkly. weight loss	2	2	2¼	2½	2½	2¼	2¾
Age 60–69:							
Select diet	D	D	D	D	E	E	F
Expected wkly. weight loss	1¼	1½	1½	1¾	1¼	1¾	1¾
Age 70–79:							
Select diet	C	D	D	D	D	–	–
Expected wkly. weight loss	1½	1	1¼	1½	1½	–	–

DIET SELECTION CHART

(and expected weekly weight loss)

MEN <u>5</u> Ft. <u>9</u> In.

If you are overweight by:

	20 lbs.	40 lbs.	60 lbs.	80 lbs.	100 lbs.	150 lbs.	200 lbs.
Age 18–19:							
Select diet	D	D	E	E	E	F	G
Expected wkly. weight loss	3½	3¾	3¼	3½	3½	3½	3½
Age 20–29:							
Select diet	D	D	D	D	D	E	E
Expected wkly. weight loss	2¾	3	3	3¼	3½	3¼	3½
Age 30–39:							
Select diet	D	D	D	D	D	D	E
Expected wkly. weight loss	2½	2½	2¾	3	3	3½	3¼
Age 40–49:							
Select diet	D	D	D	D	D	D	E
Expected wkly. weight loss	2¼	2¼	2½	2¾	2¾	3¼	3
Age 50–59:							
Select diet	D	D	D	D	D	E	E
Expected wkly. weight loss	2	2¼	2¼	2½	2¾	2½	2¾
Age 60–69:							
Select diet	D	D	D	D	E	E	F
Expected wkly. weight loss	1¼	1½	1½	1¾	1½	1¾	1¾
Age 70–79:							
Select diet	D	D	D	D	D	–	–
Expected wkly. weight loss	1	1¼	1¼	1½	1¾	–	–

DIET SELECTION CHART

(and expected weekly weight loss)

MEN 5 Ft. 10 In.

	If you are overweight by:						
	20 lbs.	40 lbs.	60 lbs.	80 lbs.	100 lbs.	150 lbs.	200 lbs.
Age 18–19:							
Select diet	D	E	E	E	E	F	G
Expected wkly. weight loss	3¾	3¼	3½	3½	3¾	3¾	3¾
Age 20–29:							
Select diet	D	D	D	D	D	E	E
Expected wkly. weight loss	3	3	3¼	3½	3½	3¼	3¾
Age 30–39:							
Select diet	D	D	D	D	D	D	E
Expected wkly. weight loss	2½	2¾	3	3	3¼	3½	3½
Age 40–49:							
Select diet	D	D	D	D	D	D	E
Expected wkly. weight loss	2¼	2½	2½	2¾	3	3¼	3
Age 50–59:							
Select diet	D	D	D	D	D	E	F
Expected wkly. weight loss	2¼	2¼	2½	2½	2¾	2½	2½
Age 60–69:							
Select diet	D	D	D	E	E	F	F
Expected wkly. weight loss	1½	1¾	1¾	1½	1½	1½	2
Age 70–79:							
Select diet	D	D	D	D	D	–	–
Expected wkly. weight loss	1¼	1¼	1½	1½	1¾	–	–

DIET SELECTION CHART

(and expected weekly weight loss)

MEN <u>5</u> Ft. <u>11</u> In.

	\multicolumn{7}{c}{If you are overweight by:}						
	20 lbs.	40 lbs.	60 lbs.	80 lbs.	100 lbs.	150 lbs.	200 lbs.
Age 18–19:							
Select diet	E	E	E	E	F	G	H
Expected wkly. weight loss	3¼	3½	3½	3¾	3½	3½	3½
Age 20–29:							
Select diet	D	D	D	D	D	E	F
Expected wkly. weight loss	3	3¼	3½	3½	3¾	3½	3½
Age 30–39:							
Select diet	D	D	D	D	D	D	E
Expected wkly. weight loss	2¾	3	3	3¼	3½	3¾	3½
Age 40–49:							
Select diet	D	D	D	D	D	D	E
Expected wkly. weight loss	2½	2½	2¾	3	3	3½	3¼
Age 50–59:							
Select diet	D	D	D	D	E	E	F
Expected wkly. weight loss	2¼	2½	2½	2¾	2¼	2¾	2¾
Age 60–69:							
Select diet	D	D	E	E	E	F	F
Expected wkly. weight loss	1½	1¾	1¼	1½	1½	1½	2
Age 70–79:							
Select diet	D	D	D	D	E	–	–
Expected wkly. weight loss	1¼	1½	1½	1¾	1¼	–	–

DIET SELECTION CHART
(*and expected weekly weight loss*)

MEN 6 Ft. 0 In.

	If you are overweight by:						
	20 lbs.	40 lbs.	60 lbs.	80 lbs.	100 lbs.	150 lbs.	200 lbs.
Age 18–19:							
Select diet	E	E	E	F	F	G	H
Expected wkly. weight loss	3½	3½	3¾	3½	3¾	3¾	3¾
Age 20–29:							
Select diet	D	D	D	D	E	E	F
Expected wkly. weight loss	3¼	3½	3½	3¾	3¼	3¾	3¾
Age 30–39:							
Select diet	D	D	D	D	D	E	E
Expected wkly. weight loss	3	3	3¼	3¼	3½	3¼	3¾
Age 40–49:							
Select diet	D	D	D	D	D	E	E
Expected wkly. weight loss	2½	2¾	2¾	3	3¼	3	3¼
Age 50–59:							
Select diet	D	D	D	D	E	E	F
Expected wkly. weight loss	2½	2½	2¾	2¾	2½	2¾	2¾
Age 60–69:							
Select diet	D	D	E	E	E	F	F
Expected wkly. weight loss	1¾	1¾	1½	1½	1¾	1¾	2
Age 70–79:							
Select diet	D	D	D	E	E	–	–
Expected wkly. weight loss	1¼	1½	1½	1¼	1¼	–	–

DIET SELECTION CHART

(and expected weekly weight loss)

MEN   6 Ft. 1 In.

	If you are overweight by:						
	20 lbs.	40 lbs.	60 lbs.	80 lbs.	100 lbs.	150 lbs.	200 lbs.
Age 18–19:							
Select diet	E	E	F	F	F	G	H
Expected wkly. weight loss	3½	3¾	3½	3¾	3¾	3¾	3¾
Age 20–29:							
Select diet	D	D	D	E	E	F	G
Expected wkly. weight loss	3½	3½	3¾	3¼	3½	3½	3½
Age 30–39:							
Select diet	D	D	D	D	D	E	F
Expected wkly. weight loss	3	3¼	3¼	3½	3¾	3½	3½
Age 40–49:							
Select diet	D	D	D	D	D	E	E
Expected wkly. weight loss	2¾	2¾	3	3	3¼	3	3½
Age 50–59:							
Select diet	D	D	D	E	E	F	G
Expected wkly. weight loss	2½	2¾	2¾	2½	2½	2½	2½
Age 60–69:							
Select diet	D	D	E	E	E	F	G
Expected wkly. weight loss	1¾	2	1½	1¾	1¾	1¾	1¾
Age 70–79:							
Select diet	D	D	D	E	E	–	–
Expected wkly. weight loss	1½	1½	1¾	1¼	1½	–	–

DIET SELECTION CHART

(and expected weekly weight loss)

MEN 6 Ft. 2 In.

	If you are overweight by:						
	20 lbs.	40 lbs.	60 lbs.	80 lbs.	100 lbs.	150 lbs.	200 lbs.
Age 18–19:							
Select diet	E	F	F	F	G	H	I
Expected wkly. weight loss	3¾	3½	3¾	3¾	3½	3½	3½
Age 20–29:							
Select diet	D	D	D	E	E	F	G
Expected wkly. weight loss	3½	3¾	3¾	3½	3½	3½	3½
Age 30–39:							
Select diet	D	D	D	D	D	E	F
Expected wkly. weight loss	3¼	3¼	3½	3¾	3¾	3½	3½
Age 40–49:							
Select diet	D	D	D	D	D	E	E
Expected wkly. weight loss	2¾	3	3	3¼	3½	3¼	3½
Age 50–59:							
Select diet	D	D	D	E	E	F	G
Expected wkly. weight loss	2½	2¾	3	2½	2¾	2¾	2¾
Age 60–69:							
Select diet	D	E	E	E	F	F	G
Expected wkly. weight loss	2	1½	1½	1¾	1½	2	2
Age 70–79:							
Select diet	D	D	E	E	E	–	–
Expected wkly. weight loss	1½	1¾	1¼	1½	1½	–	–

DIET SELECTION CHART

(*and expected weekly weight loss*)

MEN <u>6</u> Ft. <u>3</u> In.

	If you are overweight by:						
	20 lbs.	40 lbs.	60 lbs.	80 lbs.	100 lbs.	150 lbs.	200 lbs.
Age 18–19:							
Select diet	F	F	F	G	G	H	I
Expected wkly. weight loss	3½	3¾	3¾	3½	3¾	3¾	3¾
Age 20–29:							
Select diet	D	E	E	E	F	F	G
Expected wkly. weight loss	3¾	3¼	3½	3½	3¼	3¾	3¾
Age 30–39:							
Select diet	D	D	D	E	E	E	F
Expected wkly. weight loss	3¼	3½	3¾	3¼	3½	3¾	3¾
Age 40–49:							
Select diet	D	D	D	D	D	E	E
Expected wkly. weight loss	3	3	3¼	3¼	3½	3¼	3¾
Age 50–59:							
Select diet	D	D	E	E	E	F	G
Expected wkly. weight loss	2¾	3	2½	2½	2¾	2¾	2¾
Age 60–69:							
Select diet	E	E	F	F	F	G	H
Expected wkly. weight loss	1½	1¾	1½	1¾	1¾	1¾	1¾
Age 70–79:							
Select diet	D	D	E	E	E	–	–
Expected wkly. weight loss	1½	1¾	1¼	1½	1¾	–	–

Here are the diets—A through I. Read yours carefully and then turn to the explanation which follows. After all, if you are going to diet intelligently, you must understand the principles upon which the diets are based.

DIET A

BREAKFAST

4 oz. orange or grapefruit juice
or
1 whole orange or ½ grapefruit

1 egg (boiled or poached)
or
2 oz. cottage cheese

1 slice of thin-sliced bread
Beverage

MID-MORNING

If you wish, you may have:
Tea or coffee

LUNCH

If you wish, you may start with
   clear soup
or
   4 oz. tomato juice
4 oz. (½ cup) cottage cheese
or
2 oz. fish (fresh or canned without
   oil), poultry, or meat
or
1 oz. hard cheese

1 slice of bread
or
½ cup cooked vegetable

May have green salad
Dessert: None
Beverage

AFTERNOON

If you wish, you may have:
1 glass of skim milk at this time

DINNER

If you wish, you may start with
   clear soup
or
   4 oz. tomato juice
4 oz. fish, poultry, or meat
1 or 2 portions cooked vegetables
May have green salad
Bread: None
1 portion of fruit
Beverage

EVENING

If you wish, you may have:
1 glass of skim milk at this time,
or you may take your evening
dessert now instead of with
dinner

BUTTER OR OLEOMARGARINE: None   SUGAR: None

MILK:
Should have two 8-oz. glasses skim or fat-free buttermilk daily.
Must have one 8-oz. glass skim or fat-free buttermilk daily.
Once in a while, in place of 1 glass of milk *and* 1 fruit portion, you may
have one small scoop (4 oz.) of ice cream or ice milk.

DIET B

BREAKFAST
4 oz. orange or grapefruit juice
or
1 whole orange or ½ grapefruit

1 egg (boiled or poached)
or
2 oz. cottage cheese

1 slice of thin-sliced bread
Beverage

MID-MORNING
If you wish, you may have:
Tea or coffee

LUNCH
If you wish, you may start with
  clear soup
or
  4 oz. tomato juice
4 oz. (½ cup) cottage cheese
or
2 oz. fish (fresh or canned without
  oil), poultry, or meat
or
1 oz. hard cheese

1 slice of bread
or
½ cup cooked vegetable

May have green salad
Dessert: None
Beverage

AFTERNOON
If you wish, you may have:
  1 glass of skim milk at this time

DINNER
If you wish, you may start with
  clear soup
or
  4 oz. tomato juice
6 oz. fish, poultry, or meat
1 or 2 portions cooked vegetables
May have green salad
Bread: None
1 portion of fruit
Beverage

EVENING
If you wish, you may have:
  1 glass of skim milk at this time,
  or you may take your evening
  dessert now instead of with
  dinner

BUTTER OR OLEOMARGARINE: None   SUGAR: None

MILK:
Should have two 8-oz. glasses skim or fat-free buttermilk daily.
Must have one 8-oz. glass skim or fat-free buttermilk daily.
Once in a while, in place of 1 glass of milk *and* 1 fruit portion, you may
have one small scoop (4 oz.) of ice cream or ice milk.

DIET C

BREAKFAST
4 oz. orange or grapefruit juice
or
1 whole orange or ½ grapefruit

1 egg (boiled or poached)
or
2 oz. cottage cheese

1 slice of thin-sliced bread
Beverage

MID-MORNING
If you wish, you may have:
Tea or coffee

LUNCH
If you wish, you may start with
clear soup
or
4 oz. tomato juice
5 to 6 oz. (⅔ cup) cottage cheese
or
3 oz. fish (fresh or canned without
oil), poultry, or meat
or
1½ oz. hard cheese

1 slice of bread
or
½ cup cooked vegetable

May have green salad
Dessert: None
Beverage

AFTERNOON
If you wish, you may have:
1 portion of fruit
or
2 oz. cottage cheese

DINNER
If you wish, you may start with
clear soup
or
4 oz. tomato juice
6 oz. fish, poultry, or meat
1 or 2 portions cooked vegetables
May have green salad
Bread: None
1 portion of fruit
Beverage

EVENING
If you wish, you may have:
1 portion of fruit
or
2 oz. cottage cheese
or
¾ oz. hard cheese

BUTTER OR OLEOMARGARINE: None   SUGAR: None

MILK:
Should have two 8-oz. glasses skim or fat-free buttermilk daily.
Must have one 8-oz. glass skim or fat-free buttermilk daily.
Once in a while, in place of 1 glass of milk *and* 1 fruit portion, you may
have one small scoop (4 oz.) of ice cream or ice milk.

DIET D

BREAKFAST
4 oz. orange or grapefruit juice
or
1 whole orange or ½ grapefruit

1 egg (boiled or poached)
or
2 oz. cottage cheese

1 slice of thin-sliced bread
Beverage: Tea or coffee

MID-MORNING
If you wish, you may have:
Tea or coffee

LUNCH
If you wish, you may start with
clear soup
or
4 oz. tomato juice
6 oz. (¾ cup) cottage cheese
or
4 oz. fish (fresh or canned without
oil), poultry, or meat
or
2 oz. hard cheese

2 slices of bread
or
1 cup cooked vegetable
or
1 slice of bread and ½ cup cooked
vegetable

May have green salad
Dessert: 1 portion of fruit
Beverage: Tea or coffee

AFTERNOON
If you wish, you may have:
1 portion of fruit
or
2 oz. cottage cheese

DINNER
If you wish, you may start with
clear soup

or
4 oz. tomato juice
8 oz. fish, poultry, or meat
1 or 2 portions cooked vegetables
May have green salad
Bread: None
1 portion of fruit
Beverage

EVENING
If you wish, you may have:
1 portion of fruit
or
2 oz. cottage cheese
or
¾ oz. hard cheese

BUTTER OR OLEOMARGARINE: None   SUGAR: None
MILK:
Should have two 8-oz. glasses skim or fat-free buttermilk daily.
Must have one 8-oz. glass skim or fat-free buttermilk daily.
Once in a while, in place of 1 glass of milk *and* 1 fruit portion, you may
have one small scoop (4 oz.) of ice cream or ice milk.

DIET E

BREAKFAST
4 oz. orange or grapefruit juice
or
1 whole orange or ½ grapefruit

1 egg (boiled or poached)
or
2 oz. cottage cheese

1 slice of regular-sliced bread
or
½ cup cereal

Beverage

MID-MORNING
If you wish, you may have:
Tea or coffee

LUNCH
If you wish, you may start with clear soup
or
4 oz. tomato juice
8 oz. (1 cup) cottage cheese
or
6 oz. fish (fresh or canned without oil), poultry, or meat
or
3 oz. hard cheese

4 slices of bread
or
1 cup cooked vegetable and 2 slices of bread

May have green salad
Dessert: 1 portion of fruit
Beverage:

AFTERNOON
If you wish, you may have:
1 portion of fruit
or
2 oz. cottage cheese

DINNER
If you wish, you may start with clear soup
or
4 oz. tomato juice
8 oz. fish, poultry, or meat
1 or 2 portions cooked vegetables
May have green salad
Bread: None
1 portion of fruit
Beverage

EVENING
If you wish, you may have:
1 portion of fruit
or
2 oz. cottage cheese
or
¾ oz. hard cheese

BUTTER OR OLEOMARGARINE: None   SUGAR: None
MILK:
Should have two 8-oz. glasses skim or fat-free buttermilk daily.
Must have one 8-oz. glass skim or fat-free buttermilk daily.
Once in a while, in place of 1 glass of milk *and* 1 fruit portion, you **may** have one small scoop (4 oz.) of ice cream or ice milk.

BREAKFAST
4 oz. orange or grapefruit juice
or
1 whole orange or ½ grapefruit

2 eggs (boiled or poached)
or
4 oz. cottage cheese

2 slices of thin-sliced bread
or
1 cup cereal

Beverage

MID-MORNING
If you wish, you may have:
Tea or coffee

LUNCH
If you wish, you may start with clear soup
or
    4 oz. tomato juice
8 oz. (1 cup) cottage cheese
or
6 oz. fish (fresh or canned without oil), poultry, or meat
or
3 oz. hard cheese

4 slices of bread
or
1 cup cooked vegetable and 2 slices of bread

May have green salad
Dessert: 1 portion of fruit
Beverage

AFTERNOON
If you wish, you may have:
1 portion of fruit
or
2 oz. cottage cheese

DINNER
If you wish, you may start with clear soup
or
    4 oz. tomato juice
8 oz. fish, poultry, or meat
1 or 2 portions cooked vegetables
May have green salad
1 slice of bread
1 portion of fruit
Beverage

EVENING
If you wish, you may have:
1 portion of fruit
or
2 oz. cottage cheese
or
¾ oz. hard cheese

BUTTER OR OLEOMARGARINE: None   SUGAR: None
MILK:
Should have two 8-oz. glasses skim or fat-free buttermilk daily.
Must have one 8-oz. glass skim or fat-free buttermilk daily.
Once in a while, in place of 1 glass of milk *and* 1 fruit portion, you may have one small scoop (4 oz.) of ice cream or ice milk.

DIET G

BREAKFAST

4 oz. orange or grapefruit juice
or
1 whole orange or ½ grapefruit

2 eggs (boiled or poached)
or
4 oz. cottage cheese

2 slices of thin-sliced bread
or
1 cup cereal

Beverage

MID-MORNING

If you wish, you may have:
Tea or coffee

LUNCH

If you wish, you may start with
  clear soup
or
  4 oz. tomato juice
8 oz. (1 cup) cottage cheese
or
6 oz. fish (fresh or canned without
  oil), poultry, or meat
or
3 oz. hard cheese
4 slices of bread
or
1 cup cooked vegetable and 2 slices
  of bread

May have green salad
Dessert: 1 portion of fruit
Beverage

AFTERNOON

If you wish, you may have:
  1 portion of fruit
or
  2 oz. cottage cheese

DINNER

If you wish, you may start with
  clear soup
or
  4 oz. tomato juice
10 oz. fish, poultry, or meat
1 or 2 portions cooked vegetables
May have green salad
1 slice of bread
1 portion of fruit
Beverage

EVENING

If you wish, you may have:
  1 portion of fruit
and
  2 oz. cottage cheese or ¾ oz.
  hard cheese

BUTTER OR OLEOMARGARINE: None   SUGAR: None
MILK:
Should have two 8-oz. glasses skim or fat-free buttermilk daily.
Must have one 8-oz. glass skim or fat-free buttermilk daily.
Once in a while, in place of 1 glass of milk *and* 1 fruit portion, you may
have one small scoop (4 oz.) of ice cream or ice milk.

101

DIET H

BREAKFAST
6 oz. orange or grapefruit juice
or
1½ whole oranges or ½ grapefruit

2 eggs (boiled or poached)
or
4 oz. cottage cheese

2 slices of thin-sliced bread
or
1 cup cereal

Beverage

MID-MORNING
If you wish, you may have:
Tea or coffee

LUNCH
If you wish, you may start with
clear soup
or
4 oz. tomato juice
8 oz. (1 cup) cottage cheese
or
6 oz. fish (fresh or canned without
oil), poultry, or meat
or
3 oz. hard cheese

4 slices of bread
or
1 cup cooked vegetable and 2 slices
of bread

May have green salad
Dessert: 1 portion of fruit
Beverage

AFTERNOON
If you wish, you may have:
1 portion of fruit
or
2 oz. cottage cheese

DINNER
If you wish, you may start with
clear soup
or
4 oz. tomato juice
12 oz. fish, poultry, or meat
1 or 2 portions cooked vegetables
May have green salad
1 slice of bread
1 portion of fruit
Beverage

EVENING
If you wish, you may have:
1 portion of fruit
and
2 oz. cottage cheese or ¾ oz.
hard cheese

BUTTER OR OLEOMARGARINE: None   SUGAR: None
MILK:
Should have three 8-oz. glasses skim or fat-free buttermilk daily.
Must have one 8-oz. glass skim or fat-free buttermilk daily.
Once in a while, in place of 1 glass of milk *and* 1 fruit portion, you may
have one small scoop (4 oz.) of ice cream or ice milk.

102

DIET I

BREAKFAST
8 oz. orange or grapefruit juice
or
1½ oranges or ½ grapefruit

2 eggs (boiled or poached)
or
4 oz. cottage cheese

2 slices of thin-sliced bread
or
1 cup cereal

Beverage

MID-MORNING
If you wish, you may have:
Tea or coffee

LUNCH
If you wish, you may start with
clear soup
or
4 oz. tomato juice
8 oz. (1 cup) cottage cheese
or
6 oz. fish (fresh or canned without
oil), poultry, or meat
or
3 oz. hard cheese

4 slices of bread
or
1 cup cooked vegetable and 2 slices
of bread

May have green salad
Dessert: 1 portion of fruit
Beverage

AFTERNOON
If you wish, you may have:
1 portion of fruit
and
2 oz. cottage cheese

DINNER
If you wish, you may start with
clear soup
or
4 oz. tomato juice
12 oz. fish, poultry, or meat
1 or 2 portions cooked vegetables
May have green salad
2 slices of bread
1 portion of fruit
Beverage

EVENING
If you wish, you may have:
1 portion of fruit
and
2 oz. cottage cheese or ¾ oz.
hard cheese

BUTTER OR OLEOMARGARINE: None   SUGAR: None
MILK:
Should have three 8-oz. glasses skim or fat-free buttermilk daily.
Must have two 8-oz. glasses skim or fat-free buttermilk daily.
Once in a while, in place of 1 glass of milk *and* 1 fruit portion, you may
have one small scoop (4 oz.) of ice cream or ice milk.

Now I will explain these diets exactly as I do in my office—just as though you were sitting across the desk from me. I tell my patients that no question is too small, none too insignificant. Therefore do not be surprised at the details. As I shall say over and over again, the details will ultimately make the difference between success and failure.

BREAKFAST

The diet starts with breakfast even if your day starts at noon. Some people like breakfast; others do not. On this diet, you *must* have breakfast. It is one of the pillars needed to build a house of sound weight reduction. You need breakfast if your diet is to be a success. If your rebuttal is that you do not have time for breakfast, make time. Get up ten minutes earlier. Or get to work later, if you can. But don't use time as your excuse.

When they first read their breakfast menu, many of my patients shake their heads and say, "Too much food! I'll never lose." But a few weeks later, as they are losing weight, they admit they've been converted to eating breakfast.

Now let's see what constitutes a breakfast. Breakfast begins with either:

Orange or grapefruit juice

or

A whole orange or ½ of a small grapefruit

One of the first questions is how much juice? The portion is of course given on your diet sheet, but it is important to know how to determine this amount. Juice glasses contain anywhere from 3 to 6 ounces. The more a glass is flared at the top, the more difficult it is to judge its volume. So, measure your juice in a measuring cup: if you don't have one, buy one! You might take a cue from some of my patients: after you know the proper measurement, mark your juice glass and then use the same one each day. If you have breakfast in a restaurant, do not worry: it is unusual for a restaurant to serve more than 4 ounces if you order a "small" glass of juice.

The juice may be fresh, frozen, or canned—as long as no sugar has been added. Read the label!

Remember that you are limited to orange or grapefruit juice for breakfast. Why did I forbid you prune juice? Because it has *twice* the amount of calories! And if you choose a sliced orange or a half grapefruit instead, don't forget your portion control: stick to the medium-sized oranges and the small grapefruit. You already know you can't sweeten your grapefruit with sugar, but don't try to substitute honey: it is a form of sugar and so is strictly forbidden. You may use an artificial sweetener if you find that you need it. A good trick is to put a drop of liquid sweetener in a teaspoon of water and then spread the mixture over the grapefruit.

By the way, you may use artificial sweeteners (available not only in liquid but in tablet and granular form) in place of sugar for any of your foods or beverages. You may use them in cooking, too, but don't cook with saccharin because it is not heat stable. Heat will cause a chemical breakdown which gives saccharin what many people call a metallic taste. For cooking, try sodium cyclamate or calcium cyclamate (Sucaryl), since it will not decompose when exposed to heat. Sucaryl is the sweetener used in most "low-caloric" canned foods and beverages. It is safe for most people when used in reasonable quantities.

As I explained before giving you your diet, every one of your meals is based on a protein, preferably animal protein. So breakfast is no exception: you must have protein at breakfast. The breakfast protein on your diet is *either* egg or cottage cheese—in the amount specified. The egg may be boiled (very soft, very hard, or anywhere in between), or poached. You can poach either by dropping the egg (without the shell) into boiling water or by using a poacher. If you use a poacher, remember that you cannot use any butter or margarine. If the egg sticks to the pan, scrape it off as well as you can; steel wool will do the rest of the work. Some people fry an egg simply by putting it on a *very hot* skillet without butter. Again, it may stick a little, but steel wool can do the cleaning. If you have one of the specially coated pans designed for frying without butter, you can fry or scramble an egg. Or, if you like, make butterless French toast in your special frying pan: simply soak your breakfast bread portion in a beaten egg.

Not many people know that cottage cheese is an excellent *breakfast* food. You may have it creamed if you wish, but again only in the exact amount allowed in your diet plan. Inasmuch as cottage cheese is usually packaged in 8-ounce cups (read the label on your container to make certain), if you divide the cup into four parts, you will have 2-ounce portions. So don't use tablespoons to measure cottage cheese; divide the cup into quarters with a knife—and you will have no measurement problems.

If you refuse to eat eggs or cottage cheese then you may substitute *one* of the following for 1 egg or 2 ounces of cottage cheese:

¾ ounce "hard" cheese

or

1 ounce meat, poultry, or fish

Once or twice a week, you may substitute a cereal (hot or cold) for your eggs or cottage cheese, but if you do:

1) Use only *skim* milk from your daily milk allowance.
2) Omit butter.
3) Omit sugar.
4) Omit toast (usually given with breakfast).
5) And in no event choose a sugar-coated cold cereal.

Though cereals vary in their calorie content, consider ½ cup of cooked cereal as a portion, and ¾ of an individual box as a cold cereal serving.

Unless you have cereal, you *must* have bread—as many slices as are listed in your diet plan. Even if you feel you do not need it, or will be stuffed, you *must* have it. I prefer that you use the whole grain or the enriched breads which help you meet your vitamin requirements. Few other breads have the desired vitamin content, and some add unnecessary fats and carbohydrates (sugar and starches). At home your bread *must* be thin-sliced; check the wrapper.

If you are away from home at breakfast and are unable to get thin-sliced bread, take ½ to ⅔ of a regular slice. *Throw away the rest.* Make believe it dropped on the floor or fell into a dirty ash tray. If necessary, carry a dirty ash tray with you at all times! Remember, attention to the little details will spell the difference between dieting success and failure.

And while you are remembering, keep firmly in mind that your bread must not be decorated with butter, oleomargarine —did you know that there are just as many calories in oleo-margarine as in butter?—jam, jelly, preserves, marmalade, or even dietetic jam or jelly. Yours is dry bread or toast. All that you are allowed to put on it is the egg or cottage cheese you are having for breakfast. (But don't put cottage cheese on your toast the day you are having an egg.)

Difficult? We admitted dieting is difficult. It's up to you to decide whether it is worth it. Is eating your only pleasure? How important is that pat of butter to you? Look in your mirror and make up your own mind.

The next breakfast item I wish to discuss is the beverage. First of all, rule out cocoa and hot chocolate. Now as to tea, coffee, and Sanka: within the bounds of reason, you may have all you wish—hot or iced, regular or instant. I often tell my patients that they may "float in it" if they so desire. You may add lemon freely to tea—and to coffee (espresso style). But you may not add milk or cream—not even skim milk. The coffee *must* be black. Yes, black! Why? Because tea and coffee are your "escape valves": if you are to have them freely, they must be non-caloric. If you accept my black-coffee edict with pain and/or disgust, I will not be surprised, but after a while *you* will be: over 90 per cent of my patients who were accustomed to milk or cream in their coffee now agree with me that if you make yourself drink black coffee for twenty-one days, by the twenty-second day you will no longer enjoy coffee any way but black. You will probably even get finicky about brands. You see black coffee opens up a different taste world for many people.

Of course, if you drink tea for twenty-one days to avoid coffee, you will not like black coffee any better on the twenty-second day. Stick with the black coffee for three weeks. You can hate me for the whole time, but you will probably like black coffee by the twenty-second day.

You may of course use artificial sweeteners—but no sugar. Use the liquid sweeteners for iced tea or coffee.

Perhaps this is the appropriate time to discuss that delightful institution known as the morning coffee break. The rules are the same whether you have yours at home, send the office messenger out for some, or take a five-minute trip to the corner drugstore. You may have all the coffee you want—but it must be black. And you may not have anything to eat with it. If you are the type of person who cannot hold a cup of coffee in one hand without having something in the other hand, then the only thing you can do is hold two cups of coffee, one in each hand, and drink them both at the same time if you wish.

LUNCH

The best way to start on the details of lunch is with the main course: the protein. The choices are:

COTTAGE CHEESE. Otherwise known as the dieter's mainstay. Why? It is low in calories and high in volume, tasty, high in protein and calcium—a chewable dairy product low in fat. There are various kinds of cottage cheese, all of which are basically skimmed milk (no fat) products. In order to improve the taste, many of the milk companies add a very small amount of butterfat to make *creamed* cottage cheese. There is, as I explained when dealing with breakfast, no objection to creamed cottage cheese as long as you watch the portion control. As to the type of curd (small, large, pot, etc.), the choice is yours. But the amount is governed by your diet sheet.

How do you judge the number of ounces in cottage cheese served you in a restaurant? It is usually apportioned with an ice-cream scoop. A medium scoop holds an average of 4 ounces, a large scoop about 6 ounces. The cheese you buy for home, as I told you, usually comes in 8-ounce waxed containers, and so if you simply cut it into quarters while it is in the container, you will have 2-ounce portions.

FISH, SHELLFISH, POULTRY, OR MEAT. Now that you know what you can and cannot eat, your main question is undoubtedly how to meet the portion control requirements. You may well say, as most of my patients do, "It is easy for you to tell me to use 4 ounces, or 6 ounces, or whatever, but I don't know what a 4- or 6- or 8-ounce portion looks like!"

There are four ways to determine sizes, but first of all bear in mind that I am talking about weight *after* cooking, not before: meat will shrink about 20 per cent after cooking, and so you may buy one-fifth more meat than the diet specifies. I am also talking about lean cuts only. And *all* visible fat must be trimmed away: lose a little meat with the fat rather than keep a little fat with the meat.

Now for those methods of measuring portions:

1) If you buy prepackaged meat, the weight is marked on the label. If you order from a butcher, simply ask him: the butcher isn't in business to give you more than you pay for.

2) A system that works for many is to visualize one slice of sandwich white bread. Meat cut to the identical size of this bread slice would weigh 8 ounces. Thus, if you are to have a 4-ounce meat portion, the piece should be the size of half a slice of sandwich bread. And you can determine other fractions with similar ease. This method will prove particularly helpful in restaurants. And in fact once you master this way of measuring, you can determine the size of meat anywhere you are. Simply use your mind's eye.

3) If you are still in doubt—and are at home—there is always the most precise way, and that is to weigh the meat. Many of my patients prefer to do this. The best scale for this purpose is *not* a household scale but a postage scale. It is the most accurate for measuring ounces and is also less expensive than a household scale; besides, between meals it can still be used for letters.

4) Incidentally, canned fish most often comes in cans that are multiples of 3¾ ounces. Read the labels. If you are entitled to only 3 ounces, divide the can into four quarters, take three of them as your portion, and forfeit the rest.

HARD CHEESE. Just what is "hard cheese"? To explain, let me start with the fact that all cheeses except cottage cheese are handled with a knife: they are either spread or cut. The cheeses you spread are called "soft." These are not allowed— ever! The cheeses you cut, even if you melt them after cutting, are considered "hard." These are all allowed, and are very nice for lunch.

Common examples of hard cheese are: American, Swiss, Gruyère. How do you determine your portions? The average luncheonette's cheese sandwich contains 1½ to 2 ounces of cheese. When making your own sandwich, *read the label* on the package, and count the number of slices. Eight slices in an 8-ounce package makes the arithmetic rather simple, but watch the count, for there may be only 6 slices in an 8-ounce package or 8 slices in a 6-ounce package. If your diet calls for a 4-ounce meat portion, you can make a cheeseburger with 3 ounces of beefburger and ½ ounce of cheese; remember that ½ ounce of hard cheese is equal to 1 ounce of meat. But if you are not sure of a portion—don't have it.

EGGS. It is best to have your eggs for breakfast, but if you want them for lunch or dinner, consider two eggs as a lunch portion in place of cheese or meat. And, as at breakfast, have them boiled or poached only, unless you can fry them without fat.

BREAD AND VEGETABLES. In addition to the main protein, you are allowed bread and/or cooked vegetable, according to your diet sheet. Basically, *and at lunch only*, one slice of bread is considered equal to half a cup of cooked vegetable. You *must* have one or the other.

Remember that when you are home, you are expected to use only *thin*-sliced bread. Restaurants, though, rarely serve such bread, and so when you go out for lunch, I have no objection to your having regular bread. This means that you can order a sandwich. Of course, if you are entitled to only one slice of bread at lunch, your sandwich will have to be an open one. Since it may be difficult to get a restaurant to serve an open sandwich, why not order a regular one and take off the top piece of bread yourself? Of course, you must tell the waiter to omit both butter and mayonnaise.

If you prefer your protein in a regular meal rather than in a sandwich, you may take your bread with it. Or—as I just said—*for lunch only*, you may substitute a half cup of cooked vegetable for each slice of bread allowed. This is the so-called "businessman's lunch."

In addition, and in any amount that you wish, you may have a green salad of *uncooked* vegetables. But don't forget: no extras. No sprinkling of nuts; no small square of jello!

DESSERT. Some of the diets do not allow any desserts at all. If such is your case, lunch is over—except for your tea or coffee. Other diets allow one portion of fruit.

ADDITIONS. Perhaps this meal will sometimes not be large enough for you. If so, you can expand it, but the expansion comes at the *front* of the lunch: you may start with a small glass (4 ounces) of tomato juice or unsweetened cranberry juice. Or you may have clear soup. By "clear," I mean that if you put the soup in a glass, you could see through it. If there is one grain of rice, or of barley, or one strand of noodle in it, it is not considered clear. There are, therefore, basically 3 types of soups allowed: broth, consommé, and bouillon. But you may have as much of each as you want. Clear soup is a great filler. Enjoy it. If it is homemade, put it in the refrigerator and then skim off the fat. And incidentally, if you prefer, drink it cold.

All the diets contain some form of midafternoon snack. They vary from diet to diet, but are self-explanatory. And of course tea or black coffee is always allowed.

DINNER

Before describing dinner, let me define what I mean by the "dinner hour." For most people it is an evening meal, and only occasionally (as on holidays and Sundays) takes place at midday. For some people the reverse is true: their main dinner meal is at midday, and only occasionally in the evening. No matter which system you prefer, or which expediency requires, there should be no problem on your diet. In addition to breakfast, your diet calls for one light meal and one heavier meal. You may have *either* one in the evening, and the other at midday. But you may not take *part* of one meal and add it to the other. For example, you may not save the bread from lunch for dinner, nor decrease the dinner meat portion and add it to lunch. The dinner-lunch switch, if made, must be a complete switch, not a partial one.

At dinner, as with lunch, you have the option of starting with clear soup or 4 ounces of tomato juice or unsweetened cranberry juice. Or, and this is different from lunch, you may start with ¼ of a small cantaloupe. If you go to someone's home for dinner, you may find that the appetizer is ½ grapefruit or a shrimp cocktail. If you partake, you will have to consider the grapefruit as your dessert, or the shrimp as part of your main meat or fish course. Depending on the number and size of the shrimp, consider it as 1 or 2 ounces of your main course. If you think shrimp weighs nothing, just think how many shrimp could be mailed for a five-cent stamp.

For your dinner main course, the choice is among fish, shellfish, poultry, and meat. In general, the portions are double those allowed at lunch, but consult your diet for the *precise* amount you may have—and do not exceed it. If you are at a dinner in which two animal protein foods (fish *and* beef, veal *and* chicken, etc.) are served, you may have them in any combination as long as the total weight does not exceed your protein allowance.

In addition to the animal protein, you must have the number of portions of cooked vegetable stated in your diet. And you may, of course, add a green salad in any amount that you wish.

If you look through all the PFI diets, you will notice that very few of them allow any bread with dinner. This should not prove a hardship for you even when eating out, because fewer and fewer people serve bread at dinner. When you are in a restaurant, just overlook the bread tray.

And now for a happier note. You may have dessert. Every diet includes dessert at dinner. But remember that the dessert is defined precisely: you may have fruit and occasionally one of the special low-calorie gelatin desserts, *but not* the standard gelatin desserts (all of which contain sugar in the gelatin powder). And you may finish your meal with black coffee or tea. But if by chance someone put sugar in your coffee or tea, decide you are not thirsty!

All diets allow an evening snack. They vary according to your diet letter, but they are all self-explanatory.

MILK AND MILK PRODUCTS

MILK. Milk is an essential food on your diet, since it is high in most of the required nutrients. Each PFI diet calls for two glasses of milk daily: it is important that you drink them. If you have a pronounced dislike of milk, I will reluctanly compromise on one glass daily—but then you must have cheese in the portions and frequencies allowed in your diet.

Now for some necessary details about the milk you may have:

1) By a glass of milk I mean an 8-ounce glass. This is the usual water glass size, but measure yours first to be certain.

2) The milk must be fat-free. Fat-free milk may be labeled either as skim milk or as buttermilk, *but*, and it is a large *but*, you must read the carton label very carefully to be sure it contains the words "fat-free."

3) Buttermilk is a tasty form of skim milk, but unfortunately, many milk companies add butterfat to it. Any such buttermilk is not acceptable for this diet.

4) Very often, skim milk is called "modified." This is fine and even preferable if modified means the addition of vitamins, but if the skim milk has been modified by the addition of extra milk solids or milk protein, then you will be getting an unnecessary and unwelcome increase in calorie count. Therefore, check the labels carefully before you purchase the milk.

5) The surest way to get a "true" skim milk is to use powdered milk. It is cheaper, easy to prepare, and always has the exact calorie count you want. Always prepare it a day in advance. It tastes better if it has been mixed and refrigerated for at least six to eight hours before you drink it.

6) Some people complain that skim milk has a blue color. Don't worry about that: it is simply the result of skim milk's having no fat. After you drink it for a while, regular milk will begin to taste like cream.

7) You may have your daily quota of milk whenever you want it: with meals or between meals, during the day or in the evening; in small, frequent servings, or in one large serving. Most people like it at lunch, and in the evening as a snack. But the choice is yours, just as long as you stick to the amounts allowed.

If you wish, you may use your milk allowance in your cooking, but remember that you may not add it to your tea or coffee, since they are to be kept strictly non-caloric and thereby unlimited items on your diet. You may, though, mix your milk with some low-calorie soda, or add a drop of vanilla to it and put it in a blender to make what I call a vanilla "skim-shake." Or add a little instant coffee to get a coffee "skim-shake."

ICE CREAM. Yes, that's right, I said ice cream. Any flavor you like, but no nuts or other embellishment. It is another way to take milk. A 4-ounce portion of ice cream—the size of a small Dixie cup—may be used in place of 1 glass of milk. But you may *never* have more than 4 ounces of ice cream in one day—and never more than 3 portions in a week. Furthermore, when you do substitute a 4-ounce portion of ice cream for a glass of milk, you must also give up one of your allowed fruit portions for that day.

So, when the entire family goes out on Sunday afternoon for ice cream, you may have some too. While you are enjoying yourself, think about what a great way this is to hide the fact that you are on a diet.

ICED DESSERTS. I have often been asked the difference between ice cream, dietetic ice cream, ice milk, sherbet, and ices. They may be summarized as follows:

Ice cream: high in calories because of fat content. Fairly high amount of calcium and protein.

Dietetic ice cream: fewer calories than in ice cream. Much less sugar.

Ice milk: even fewer calories than in dietetic ice cream— and by far the best form for the dieter. It looks and tastes like ice cream, has a high amount of calcium and protein, but is made from milk instead of cream.

Milk sherbet: can be very high in calories depending on how it was made. Many have excess sugar. Varies also in the amount of milk it contains. Must be checked carefully.

Ices: composed mostly of sugar and water. Contain no protein or calcium. Therefore, ices are not allowed on your diet.

YOGURT. Since yogurt differs from milk primarily in that it is a special type of culture, it may not be used as a main course any more than you could use milk that way: it is just not a substitute for the protein needed at breakfast, lunch, and dinner. Its calorie content varies from one and a half to two times that of skim milk, depending upon the type of processing, and it is therefore not allowed as a milk substitute. If you do love it, however, you may use *unflavored* yogurt as an ice-cream substitute. (Flavored yogurts are disqualified because they contain extra calories because of the additional sugar.) Four ounces (½ cup) of yogurt equals a portion of ice cream on our diets.

ALCOHOL

Having finished with milk, let us turn to another liquid: alcohol. I am concerned here only with how alcohol affects dieting. Alcohol has five distinct disadvantages for the dieter.

1) It adds extra calories.

2) Taken in moderate amounts, it frequently increases the appetite.

3) Taken in excessive amounts, alcohol will "confuse the appetite" and make a patient lose even the most intense resolve.

4) It is often associated with high-calorie hors d'oeuvres.

5) And it is commonly associated with high-calorie mixers. Some of the tonics or quinine waters have as many calories as an equal amount of ginger ale or cola.

You cannot therefore, expect to be able to drink without limit. The amount must be rigidly controlled. Nor can you compensate by taking away food from your diet to make room for alcohol: after all, the PFI diets are based on nutrition requirements. The alcohol must be in addition to your diet. If you drink, you must be willing to lose at a slightly lesser rate than you would if you did not drink. In most instances your drinking will not affect your weight loss by more than ¼ pound per week—but little as that sounds, it represents about ⅛ (over 10 per cent) of the average anticipated weight loss each week.

And so, if at all possible, *do not drink*. And in any case, *never drink alone*: you will be satisfying no social need, which is the one reason for allowing alcohol in your diet.

If you are to drink, your alcohol intake must be considered by the same rules of portion, frequency, and item control.

PORTION CONTROL

We judge each drink according to the size of the glass in which it is usually served:

Ale or beer—8-oz. glass (not a 12-oz. bottle)
Brandy—1½-oz. jigger
Whiskey—1½-oz. jigger
Wine (except sherry)—3- to 4-oz. glass
Cordial—1-oz. glass
Sherry—2-oz. glass

Each of the above sizes is considered as *one drink* (alcohol portion). You may have your drinks in any combination, as long as you do not exceed the amount per drink or the number of drinks allotted per week.

As to *mixers*, you may use club soda (*not* sweet soda), plain water, non-caloric dietetic soda, or have your drink on the rocks (just with ice). Remember, though, that the taller the drink, the longer it should last. It is as important to drink slowly as it is to eat slowly.

FREQUENCY CONTROL

The maximum number of drinks you are allowed in one week follows. If you are not a big drinker, set yourself a lower maximum.

If you are on diets A, B, or C and your weekly weight loss is to be *less than* 2 pounds, you may not have more than 3 drinks per week.

If you are on diets A, B, or C, but your diet calls for a loss of 2 *pounds or more* weekly, you may not have more than 7 drinks per week.

If yours is diet D, E, F, G, H, or I, you may not have more than 7 drinks per week.

ITEM CONTROL

All types of alcohol are allowed (in the amounts listed) except for mixed cocktails (daiquiris, manhattans, martinis, mint juleps, old-fashioneds, planters punch, etc.) and *eggnog*.

Questions Patients Ask

WHAT DO I DO IF I GET HUNGRY OR THIRSTY DESPITE MY DIET?
I call this the HAT problem.

H-A-T stands for *h*unger *a*nd *t*hirst. Even the best planned and most carefully followed diet cannot completely avoid these obstacles. Fat or thin, all human beings are sometimes hungry and sometimes thirsty. But there is no need to panic, no need to say the diet doesn't work. Though it is true: diets *don't* work—*you* do the work!

When you are hungry, ask yourself what you would do if it were 2 P.M., you were at work, and felt sleepy. Would you just take time off for a nap? I doubt it. You would force yourself to continue working, and in time your sleepiness would disappear. Similarly, just because you are hungry, you do not have to feel that the whole world must stop revolving so that you can get something to eat. The desire to eat will often pass, particularly if you occupy yourself—especially your hands. *You can live for a little while without food!*

Besides, remember that your diet allows you between-meal snacks. Do not be afraid to have them. They will help you keep to your regimen and learn the appetite control that will result in weight maintenance. If you can do without snacks, fine, but you needn't be a Spartan to survive this diet. You will find that milk (in the portion allotted) makes an especially satisfying snack.

119

If you need additional help for hunger pangs, try the following:

1) Have as much as you want of carrots or celery, or any raw vegetable. Now, obviously, I am not suggesting that you eat 18 bunches of raw carrots or a dozen green peppers in one sitting: you don't need this book if all you are trying to do is kid yourself. But within reason, enjoy your fresh vegetable snacks.

Keep the raw vegetables, *ready to eat*, in the refrigerator. Remember, you may want something to eat late in the evening, and I doubt that you will be willing to clean, scrape, or cut vegetables at night. So prepare for the possibility by having your celery, carrots, or other raw vegetables ready ahead of time and left in the refrigerator *completely immersed in water*. They will stay crisp and fresh for weeks this way and will always be available when you want them. If they are to accompany you out of the house, wrap them in wax paper and see how easily they fit into a lunch box or pocket.

2) Have bouillon, or any other completely clear soup in any amount (unless you have high blood pressure, in which case ask your doctor first; bouillon has a very high salt content and your physician may have restricted your salt intake).

Thirst can be handled without difficulty. There is no need for most individuals to restrict their fluid intake. The following may be used in reasonably unlimited quantity.

1) Tea or black coffee—either hot or cold. It does not matter if the tea or coffee is "fresh brewed" or instant, but it must be without cream, milk, or sugar. Lemon is fine.

2) Club soda (not sweet soda). You can make lemonade by using a little fresh lemon juice (or unsweetened canned lemon juice) with club soda and an artificial sweetening agent.

3) The non-caloric sodas. There are many brands available; choose only the ones which contain almost zero calories per glass. Try putting some of the soda in a large brandy glass together with ice. It looks special this way and, for reasons

unknown to me, seems to taste better. But don't overdo the amount of these carbonated beverages; after all, you are trying to control your desire for a sweet taste.

4) The best of all is so very old fashioned a remedy that I saved it for last. Water, of course. After all, this is what controls all thirst!

DON'T I NEED PILLS? This is a question which you should discuss with your physician. But I can tell you some things about pills.

First of all, pills do not reduce your weight. Some are designed to increase your metabolic rate. These should never be taken except as prescribed by your physician. Most of the pills used for dieting are those which suppress the appetite. These, too, are potent medications, and should be taken only if your physician agrees. If he prescribes them, follow his instructions precisely, but remember, they can never be a substitute for our threesome: motivation, food education, self-discipline. I personally suggest pills rarely. In my experience, the appetite-suppression medications become a crutch that can prevent you from learning proper food habits. You cannot restrain an appetite in the absence of an appetite any more than you can teach a child to write without giving him a pencil. The pencil is the tool that must be handled, not destroyed, if the pupil is to learn to write. The appetite is the tool that must be handled, not destroyed, if the dieter is to learn to eat correctly. Again, if you avoid the word *easy* from the start, you will be on the road to success.

WHAT IF RELIGIOUS REQUIREMENTS INTERFERE WITH MY DIET? Religious customs often involve food requirements: avoidance of certain foods, or of mixing others; the use of sacramental beverages and foodstuffs; the use of special foods; as well as partial and total fasts. But most such requirements aid the cause of dieting, simply because they are restrictive. Sacramental foods and beverages are used in such small amounts that they produce no practical problems. Of course, if you drink a large goblet of wine when you are required to take only a sip, whom are you fooling? Remember: you are the one who wishes to reduce. If you fast, you may *not* change your diet either before or after the fast. If special foods are required for your religious needs, learn the equivalent for the usual foods outlined in your diet.

MAY I HAVE SALT? CAN YOU HAVE TOO MUCH WATER? WHAT ABOUT SPICES? If you have high blood pressure, a peptic ulcer, kidney disease, or other diseases requiring a physician's care, he will advise you on the proper amount of salt and water allowed for dietary purposes. But if you are in perfect health, except for being overweight, there is no need for you to restrict your salt intake. Of course, the amount of salt you use will control your degree of thirst and in turn both your water intake and water retention. But after all, salt and water are essential for life. If your body organs are normal, you will always be in balance between the faucet and bathroom. So let your taste and thirst be your guide as to salt and water intake.

Occasionally, heavy salt users do show some water retention. This is what I call "water weight," but since it does not interfere with fat loss, it is no real problem. If you appear to be a "water retainer," discuss it with your physician. Incidentally, weight reduction diets by themselves do not cause water retention, but the frequent weighing and attention to weight-loss progress makes water retention, when present, more apparent.

Water retention is often experienced by women just before a menstrual period: weight may well go up every fourth week from this cause, but it is usually completely lost by the following week.

Again, unless you have an illness, there is no reason why you cannot use any spices freely, except those, like catsup, which contain sugar. In fact, I urge you to explore the world of herbs and spices. They can add sparkle to a repetitious routine.

MAY I HAVE PICKLES AND SAUERKRAUT? Indeed you may—as long as the pickles are not sweet. Consider pickles and sauerkraut as raw vegetables. But note that too much of either may make you temporarily retain fluids. Incidentally, make sure no sugar was added to the sauerkraut.

WHAT IS FATTENING FOOD? Too much of almost any food can make you fat! Yet you can eat the highest calorie-containing foods in proper portions and still not gain weight! I therefore avoid using the term "fattening food." A good diet provides the *right* foods for you, defines the amount that should be eaten, and prohibits the wrong foods for you. In general, the diets in this book stress those foods that have the least number of calories per portion, and recommend portion sizes based on satisfying your real needs. If you must be descriptive, use the phrase high-calorie foods or low-calorie foods; omit the term fattening.

WHAT ARE EMPTY CALORIES? The term "empty" calories is applied to those foods that offer only calories—and very little in the form of protein, minerals, or vitamins. Empty calories, wherever possible, are understandably enough avoided in the diets in this book.

Soft drinks—the various colas, soda pops, commercial "ades" and fruit drinks—are a common example of "empty calories," since they are made up of water, sugar, and flavoring. As you know, they are not allowed on your diet. If you can't quench your thirst with water, have the non-caloric soft drinks in reasonable amounts.

WHY ARE SOME DIETETIC FOODS ALLOWED AND OTHERS NOT? The answer is that there is a variety of dietetic foods on the market; I am sure that at times it seems as though all packaged foods are "dietetic." Just remember that the labels on the packages are all-important, because the term may mean something different to each manufacturer. Dietetic foods have one or all of the following characteristics:

1) Simple calorie reduction—most often accomplished by a reduction in absorbable fat. This calorie reduction may

be small or quite significant. Salad dressings are good examples of both extremes.

2) Calorie reduction achieved by omitting syrup and replacing sugar with artificial sweetening agents. Many dietetic fruits are in this group.

3) Calorie reduction accomplished by replacement of syrup with plain water. These foods are usually labeled "water-packed."

4) Calorie reduction by omitting oil—as in some of the canned fishes.

5) Reduction in sugar *and* fats, as in dietetic cookies.

6) Reduction in calories and sodium (salt-free, low-calorie foods).

7) Reduction in sodium alone.

There are other so-called dietetic foods, less easily categorized. Just read their labels. If they are not carefully labeled, do not buy them. You have a right to know what you are buying.

By now, you should have memorized the fact that if you follow any of the diets listed in this book, the following dietetic foods are strictly and completely forbidden to you:

Dietetic candy
Dietetic cookies and cake
Dietetic jams, jellies, and preserves

You must stop trying to satisfy your "sweet tooth." It is unnecessary. No, I am not cruel: I am simply interested in your diet being successful.

ALL RIGHT, THEN, HOW DO YOU STOP A CRAVING FOR SWEETS? The most effective food to counteract such a craving is a *sour pickle*! Try it. It works!

I must admit I suggested a different technique to one patient of mine, a woman who seemed to live from one sweet taste to the next. Janet P. had been fat since childhood but "this time" was determined to lose weight. She started her diet eagerly and did well at first. After a while, however, she began to beg for a sweet taste. "Not a big piece of candy," she explained, "just a taste." I, of course, said that under no circumstances could she have any candy, not even a dietetic one: first, even dietetic candies have too many calories for a PFI diet; second, and more important, the use of them would only delay her learning proper eating habits.

Mrs. P. understood my reasoning, but she couldn't hold to the practice of the theory: she was succumbing to her desires —resenting the fact, feeling guilty, but still stealing the occasional sweet.

I tried something which I have used ever since, most successfully. I advised Janet P. to carry saccharin tablets with her wherever she went: every time she felt an "uncontrollable" desire for sweets, she could put a plain saccharin tablet on her tongue and let it dissolve. I knew that the sweetness in a tablet is so concentrated that the taste would be almost sickening—and she would have a slightly bitter metallic aftertaste as well. Anyway, Mrs. P. soon discovered she was craving sweets less and less. She no longer carries saccharin with her and says that every time she wants a piece of candy she just thinks about the saccharin tablet.

WHAT ABOUT VITAMINS AND MINERALS? The diets in this book were designed to insure your getting a sufficient supply of essential vitamins and minerals: that is why I stress particularly the importance of eating enriched or whole-grain breads and of having a daily portion of citrus fruit.

Most Americans start the day with citrus fruit or juice—a wonderful habit since this is our chief source of Vitamin C. Vitamin C is essential for good health, and yet is not stored in the body; the supply must, therefore, be replenished constantly. If you are allergic to citrus fruits, ask your physician about substitute foods or Vitamin C tablets. But if your problem is simply that you do not like a cold drink first thing in the morning, *don't* heat the juice. Heat destroys Vitamin C. Instead, try having your juice after your coffee!

Now as to vitamins and minerals in relation to dieting: firstly, they neither add nor reduce weight. And there is no substantial evidence that extra vitamins will increase the appetite of an obese person. If your food is stored and prepared carefully, it should have no appreciable loss of vitamins. But even though the PFI diets contain all the necessary vitamins, it is possible that because of the food choice you are allowed, you will not achieve a perfect vitamin intake. And so I suggest that you add to your diet a vitamin preparation with the following vitamins in the approximate amounts listed.

Vitamin A	5,000 to 10,000 I.U.
Vitamin D	400 I.U.
Thiamine (B-1)	2 to 5 mg.
Riboflavin (B-2)	2 to 5 mg.
Niacinamide	10 to 30 mg.
Pyridoxine (B-6)	0.5 to 5.0 mg.
Ascorbic Acid (C)	50 to 100 mg.

Many drug firms sell vitamin preparations containing this formulation. Some are available without prescription; others require a prescription. But unless your physician specifically prescribes one of them, there is rarely a need for the extra high potency therapeutic-type preparations. They are expensive and unnecessary for most people: the water-soluble vitamins can be stored in the body only for short periods of time; excess vitamins of this type are usually excreted in the urine and wasted.

Stuffing yourself with high potency vitamins in dosages higher than that recommended rarely offers any advantages and can be potentially dangerous. There are many reports of severe problems developing from overdosages of Vitamins A and D.

There is no need for you to add mineral preparations, unless your physician prescribes them; your diet provides adequate amounts.

Be careful, too, of the "food supplements." They are often not called vitamins simply because they do not meet the government requirements for vitamins: they may lack adequate potency, or their source or way of having been manufactured may be questionable. Do not guess at reliability. You wouldn't buy a TV set without knowing about the manufacturer or the dealer, and health is more important than entertainment. Let your physician guide you on vitamin selection. Use a reliable druggist and a reliable vitamin manufacturer. There are rarely bargains when it comes to health.

WHAT IF I CATCH A COLD? I am sure that you are aware that when you have a cold, you should increase your consumption of fluids. But instead of taking fruit juices (and thereby adding calories), why not use water for the fluid and ask your doctor for a prescription for Vitamin C (ascorbic acid).

If you have a cough, don't try to treat it with honey. Honey has no medicinal value, and, since it is pure sugar, it is forbidden on your diet.

WHAT'S WRONG WITH FAD DIETS? Too many of them do not meet the requirements of good nutrition and thereby jeopardize your health. No one should try a starvation diet—the total removal of food except for non-caloric liquids—without a physician's consent. Crash diets vary in details of food intake, but they, too, may be injurious to health; besides, they are unpleasant to follow and rarely provide lasting results. Obviously, I do not recommend them.

Liquid-formula diets, on the other hand, have the advantage of giving you a precise caloric control. But they rarely meet the social needs of the dieter: can you tell the boss's wife who invited you for dinner that you are on a liquid diet? And how long can you stick to a liquid diet? They are not designed to teach you good eating habits—the kind which you can follow even after the completion of the diet. And so, though liquid diets may seem to offer the easy way, they all too often result in the perpetual weight seesaw. In addition, many who use the liquid formulas complain of gastrointestinal problems, particularly constipation and "gas."

CHAPTER 4

Preparation Hints for the Dieter

Though this is not a cookbook, I do want to try to give you some cooking and serving suggestions—many of them made by my patients. Here, then, are ways that some of the basic food-preparation problems can be handled by the cook for the benefit of the dieter whether the dieter is you or someone else in your family.

Problem 1: Since there is an over-all reduction in total food, portions appear skimpy.

Solution: Use smaller plates. I am very serious about this: an overflowing small plate will look like a lot of food!

Problem 2: These diets are repetitious. Won't they become monotonous?

Solution: Utilize all the varieties allowed. Alternate eggs with cottage cheese at breakfast, for example. Try as many of the fruits and vegetables as you can. Serve your foods attractively. Use garnishes such as parsley and watercress freely. And plan colorful meals: carrots with string beans are more appetizing than string beans with spinach. Finally, use herbs and spices liberally.

Problem 3: Extra use of spices may result in too high a salt intake for some dieters.

Solution: Avoid the salty spices (salt itself, garlic salt, onion salt, and artificial seasonings containing monosodium glutamate). Instead of using garlic or onion salt, use the flavorings in fresh or powdered form.

Problem 4: What do you do when vegetables or fruits are out of season?

Solution: There is always a good variety of seasonal fruits and vegetables available. Be a little adventuresome. With better refrigeration and transportation, the "season" for all fruits and vegetables is getting longer and longer. Canned foods are always available, but remember to make sure they do not contain sugar.

Problem 5: Some foods "really" need oils or fats to prepare them properly.

Solution: No, they don't. *Properly* is a personal word. They can be made appetizing without fat or oil. You must adjust to different tastes when dieting.

Problem 6: Some foods require breading, or use of flour.

Solution: No, they don't. See answer to Problem 5.

Problem 7: Some foods must be basted. For example, chicken broiled without fat just doesn't taste right.

Solution: As I suggested earlier you may use tomato or lemon juice, consommé or bouillon freely when broiling meat, fish, or poultry. You can try a *truly* dietetic French dressing (one with less than 3 calories per teaspoon). Or you can make a soup stock yourself, and strain through a coarse strainer. But you must follow what I call the prime cooking rule. Never baste with anything *unless* the basting substance is hot. If you use a soup stock or tomato juice, heat it before using. Cold liquids added to cooking foods draw out the natural juices, whereas heat will seal them in. (You follow the same principle when you remove bloodstains from clothing: you use cold water because you know that hot water sets the blood.)

Problem 8: How do you skim the fat off soups?

Solution: Put the soup in the refrigerator until it jells. The fat will be at the top. Cut it off, reheat, and it is ready to serve.

Problem 9: What can be used for stewing meats?

Solution: As I have said, I prefer that you broil meats and poultry over a rack so that the fat will drip off. If you do stew, however, put in *any* of the allowed vegetables you wish, as long as you follow these rules:

1) Measure the total amount of vegetables added, regardless of type.
2) If the vegetables add up to less than half a cup for the dieter's portion, he may have them in addition to his regular allotment.
3) If the vegetables add up to over half a cup (but less than one cup) for the dieter's portion, they must count as one cooked vegetable serving.
4) Make sure you remove *all* visible fat from any stewing meat *before* cooking.

Problem 10: What can the dieter eat while sitting at the table waiting for the main course to be served?

Solution: Time the meal serving carefully; the food should be ready when the dieter sits down. Also, you can serve the salad before the main course to abate hunger.

Problem 11: Is there any way of varying the salad dressing, except by using the spices and juices already mentioned?

Solution: Try the specially prepared vinegars such as tarragon vinegar or wine vinegar.

Problem 12: Are there any special tricks to cooking with milk?

Solution: Yes. Try using the dry nonfat milk powder (skim milk), but remember to deduct the milk you use from your daily allowance. (One-sixth of a cup of skim milk powder equals one 8-ounce glass of liquid milk.) For each cup of fluid milk called for in your recipe, put 3 to 4 tablespoons of the powder in 1 cup of water.

Problem 13: Can I start lunch or dinner with a fruit?

Solution: Once in a while, and only if you are allowed a fruit as dessert at that meal. Of course, you must then omit dessert.

Problem 14: Can unsweetened gelatin be used?
Solution: Yes, both for desserts and in salads.

Problem 15: May condiments similar to, but other than, catsup be used?
Solution: Yes, if used in amounts of *less* than 1 teaspoon. Mustard may be used freely, as well as Tabasco sauce, and any of the pure herbs.

Problem 16: The diet encourages fish. How does one prepare it without butter?
Solution: By steaming, boiling, baking, or broiling. Use lemon or tomato juice. Keep both juices hot. If you wrap your fish in aluminum foil, the water will stay in and keep the fish from drying out. Use a low flame. For extra flavor, try pan-broiling the fish; first brown some onions or mushrooms directly on a fat-free skillet and then place the fish on them.

Problem 17: How can you prepare steak without butter?
Solution: Easily; it doesn't need it.

Problem 18: How do you prepare veal?
Solution: Veal is a lean, short-fibered meat. Always cook it over a low flame. Keep it covered or wrapped in aluminum foil. The answer to Problem 16 is equally pertinent here.

Problem 19: What can be used for seafood sauce?
Solution: A mixture of tomato juice, horseradish, Tabasco, herbs, and spices.

Problem 20: What are the best hors d'oeuvres for the dieter?
Solution: Celery, carrots—and a desire to lose weight!

Problem 21: Are any desserts besides fruit allowed?
Solution: Yes. As I have said before, you may use the dietetic gelatin desserts. Try adding ½ portion of fruit to one. You can make your own low-calorie gelatin dessert by using an unsweetened gelatin and, in place of water, a low-calorie dietetic soda. Stir the soda first to remove the bubbles. Other desserts can be made with lemon or lime (juice and rind), artificial sweetener, egg whites, and unsweetened gelatin.

Problem 22: How do you cook a meal for dieter and non-dieter alike?

Solution: It is difficult to create hard and fast rules. Certainly, it will not hurt the rest of your family to develop good eating habits, cut down on cakes and pastries, and increase fish and poultry eating. Very often identical foods can be prepared for all members of the family, the only difference being in the portion control of the dieter. But at times, you must prepare specially. Let's face it: dieting is not easy—you must be willing to put in some extra work, whether for yourself or for another family dieter.

CHAPTER 5

Keep Your Own Records

We have now reached the point where you certainly have enough knowledge to start your diet. If you still have any questions about a specific food, *do not eat it* until you look up the answer both in your diet and in the index.

To assist you on your diet, I am suggesting two things my patients have found to be wonderful aids:

1) Get a small notebook, date each page, and write down on it every item you eat or drink—except water; how much of it and how it was prepared. Carry the notebook with you always and check it every night against your diet and the instructions in this book. If checking takes too much time, you are probably eating too much! Don't stop keeping the daily record; it will help you stick to your diet—*if* you don't leave out any details.

2) Keep a separate chart of your progress to make sure you are losing the number of pounds per week specified in your diet.

Following is a sample Achievement Chart. You will see that on the top line of the second column you write the date and in the space to its right, your weight. In the next column put in the weekly predicted weight loss according to your diet. From the first week on, fill in all entries. If you are a woman who has not undergone menopause, put in the letters M.P. (for menstrual period) if your menstruation *started* within the seven-day period preceding the current entry. Do this so that you can make allowance for the usual pattern of water retention which precedes your menstrual period (it is automatically controlled the following week).

ACHIEVEMENT CHART

End of Week	Date	Weight	Predicted Weekly Wt. Loss	Actual Wt. Loss this week	Predicted Wt. Loss so far Total	Actual Wt. Loss so far	Notes
Start	9/23	168					
1	9/30	163	—2	—5	—2	—5	M.P. (9/28)
2	10/7	160	—2	—3	—4	—8	
3	10/14	159	—2	—1	—6	—9	
4	10/21	158½	—2	—½	—8	—9½	
5	10/28	156	—2	—2½	—10	—12	M.P. (10/26)
6	11/4	154	—2	—2	—12	—14	
7	11/11	152½	—2	—1½	—14	—15½	
8	11/18	153½	—2	+1	—16	—14½	
9	11/25	149½	—2	—4	—18	—18½	M.P. (11/23)
10	12/2	147	—2	—2½	—20	—21	
11	12/9	145½	—2	—1½	—22	—22½	Changed to Diet B

Part III

CHAPTER 1

Home Dilemmas

Unquestionably, the most difficult situations faced by dieters are the social and occupational ones. And so in this section I will cover various problems involved and give examples of how some patients have handled them. But eating at home presents its own challenge, and we should begin with that.

WHY YOUR FRIEND IS FAT

Home usually means family, and family often gets the blame for overweight. And so we get to the case of the friend who says she has a fat parent, or possibly two fat parents. Also, one of her sisters is fat, so obviously her fatness must be inherited.

It is true that fat children's parents are usually fat, and that fat people bring up fat children. But does this mean that over-weight is inherited? The most detailed analysis has not so shown. There *is* a strain of mice considered to have "hereditary obesity." Yet even these mice can be made to lose weight by a simple restriction of their food.

All right, then, why is it so common for fat people to have fat parents? Where does the overweight problem really start? Probably in early childhood—at the dining table. It may not show then, but childhood is when food habits develop. If mother and father always put sugar and cream in cereal, or feel that bread and baked potatoes cannot be eaten without butter, or that a meal is not complete without cake, they undoubtedly feel that what is good for them is good for their child. And so, in my opinion, fatness in the family is a dining-table "inheritance"—not a scientific one. It need not go beyond one generation, because it is not true inheritance. It is the influence of home environment, not heredity. Your friend, then, does not have the tendency to be fat: she has the tendency to overeat! A tendency developed in the course of her growing up.

Your friend may also have the tendency to try to "eat away" her troubles, her dissatisfactions. Whatever her reason, the fact remains: it takes food to be fat! Your friend may not be willing to face the fact, but she can lose weight if she restricts her food.

Incidentally, if she reads this book, do you think she will think of *you* at this point?

THE CASE OF THE TWO LETTUCE LEAVES EATER

Mrs. L. was in her early forties. She had two children, both in college, one a freshman and the other a senior. With her children away at school, and her husband frequently off on business trips, she found there was little need for her to spend much time in the kitchen. She could participate in community activities and even take one of the new courses for adults. A busy woman, with much self-generated activity, she was nevertheless about 20 pounds overweight and had been "trying" to lose weight for years.

Mrs. L. was convinced her problem was her metabolism because all she ate was "toast and coffee for breakfast; a tiny salad and a cup of tea for lunch; meat and vegetable for dinner; never any dessert," and yet she "couldn't lost an ounce" though she ate less than her friends did! I did metabolism tests; hers was perfectly normal.

This is a familiar type of patient: we call such the "two lettuce leaves eater." Just what is the problem here? She is not a liar, but at the same time her weight doesn't come from the air. Medical science has shown beyond any doubt that if *you* eat fewer calories than you "burn," *you* must lose weight.

I gave Mrs. L. PFI Diet B, and she was quite insistent that she could not possibly lose weight with it as she ate less than the diet allowed. I was more insistent, however, and made her promise that she would follow the diet precisely, even though it was "too much to eat." Much to her surprise (and delight) she lost about 1¾ pounds per week. And though her original complaint was that the diet allotted her too much food, now she had occasional periods of hunger.

What is the explanation? Mrs. L. hadn't realized how many hidden calories she was eating. First of all, Mrs. L. was a short woman. Short people have a smaller body skin or surface area and therefore require fewer calories than do taller individuals; Mrs. L. had in fact been eating less than her friends, but she needed less. But more important was to make her realize how many calories she had been eating: pre-diet calorie intake turned out to be about 1800–1900 calories daily even though she was convinced it was less than half that. Her "toast and coffee" actually consisted of two pieces of toast—full thickness—with oleomargarine and sometimes jelly. She had two cups of coffee ("it was not fattening") with just a little milk ("little" meant approximately 1 ounce, or 20 calories) in each cup. This was preceded by 4 ounces of orange juice. All this added up to 250 to 350 calories! Her PFI breakfast consisted of:

> 4 ounces of orange juice
> 1 slice of dry toast (thinly-sliced)
> 1 egg or 2 ounces of cottage cheese
> Black coffee

This added up to 195 calories and yet was more satisfying and had more quality protein than did her previous breakfast. Furthermore, it removed her need for a cracker nibble in the late morning. And breakfast was only one example of the hidden calories in Mrs. L.'s former diet.

Mrs. L. was not a jealous person, but even she had fallen victim to the *dietary illusion* which causes the most frequent complaint of the overweight individual: "My friend eats everything. I've seen her; I've eaten with her. She doesn't gain an ounce! But I, I just look at food and get fat!"

When a patient says this to me, I explain that first of all, you are rarely able to observe a friend's eating habits 24 hours a day. But even if you were, you would have to understand food values to make a valid comparison of her meals and yours. Your drugstore lunch of a hamburger on a bun (loaded with catsup), a small slice of tomato (with a dab of mayonnaise), a small paper container of coleslaw (which usually is made with mayonnaise), coffee with a little milk and saccharin, is remembered and recounted as a luncheon consisting of "a small hamburger and coffee." Your friend who eats everything may have a cup of broth, a chicken sandwich with a slice of tomato but no butter, a small dish of ice cream, and iced tea with lemon. To you, the lunch of the thin friend seems enormous: after all, soup, sandwich, ice cream, and tea! But let us count the calories:

Your Lunch	*Calories*
Hamburger	225
Soft bun	178
Tomato catsup	30
Cole slaw (cabbage	12
made with mayonnaise—1 teaspoon)	35
Tomato slice	5
Mayonnaise (½ tablespoon)	50
Coffee with a "little" milk	20
Total Calories	555

Your Friend's Lunch	*Calories*
Broth	11
Chicken sandwich with two slices of bread	303
Tomato slice	5
Ice cream	200
Tea with lemon	4
Total Calories	523

Both calorie counts are similar but your "hardly anything" lunch actually contained 32 more calories than that of your "eat everything" friend. *Who* is just looking at food and gaining weight?

Incidentally, don't overlook that interlude during afternoon shopping. You may think you are being careful by having a baked apple without cream, while your diet-unconscious friend has a piece of packaged pound cake with black coffee. Yet a baked apple as ordinarily prepared (it is usually large and loaded with sugar) has 194 calories, while a slice of pound cake has 130 calories! Another 65-calorie difference!

The 12 o'clock lunch and 4 o'clock snack have now resulted in a difference of almost 100 calories daily between you and your friend. If this difference were maintained six days a week, there would be an 8-pound difference in body weight at the end of one year. Five years would make it 40 pounds!

If you "look at food and gain," stop looking—and start choosing! All you are seeing is the *dietary illusion.* Your friend "who eats everything" is really a better chooser.

The Breakfast Haters

Many overweight persons counter my demand for food-content awareness by saying they could save calories if I would not insist that they eat breakfast. They complain that they aren't hungry first thing in the morning.

Let's analyze this. Many overweight people are not hungry in the morning because they have not recovered from stuffing themselves during the preceding evening and night. Others would rather sleep the few extra minutes it takes to have breakfast. And still others feel that they cannot eat *immediately* after arising. The answer to the last group is to dress *completely* first, and then have breakfast. The time it takes to get dressed is often enough to allow you to develop an appetite for the meal. Have you ever noticed that when on a vacation, even non-breakfasters tend to eat a real breakfast? Part of the reason is the relaxation which comes with vacation, but there is also the factor of the time lapse between arising and getting to a restaurant or hotel dining room: time enough to whet the appetite.

Why *must* you eat breakfast? First, as I explained in detail when covering the meal, it is the foundation for the day's diet. Second, it provides the energy for the morning's activities (this has been well proven in the Iowa Breakfast Studies). Third, it helps to take you through to lunch without the temptation of nibbling.

Most overweight individuals seem to have what I call a *hidden hunger*. It is the kind of hunger that is appeased by many small bites rather than one large meal. That is why I make allowance for between-meal snacks on the diet. But in my experience the best preventive for hidden hunger is breakfast. I have learned that it is rare for the dieter to be permanently successful without the benefit of a good breakfast.

Happily, it is rare for a patient who has dieted successfully not to have become a breakfast lover. In fact, one patient told me a very interesting story. Before the diet he had never eaten breakfast, but was forced to by my insistence. After he had been on the diet for about seven weeks, he had awakened late one morning and rushed to get ready for work. He had driven halfway into the city when he realized he was just too hungry, and headed for the nearest diner. He was an additional ten minutes late to the office, but had discovered that he was now a truly confirmed breakfast eater.

The Woman Who Wouldn't Eat Rabbit Food

Mrs. K. was an attractive young woman who didn't look as though she needed to lose weight. When somebody like that comes to my office, it almost always means the same thing: a weight distribution problem. This woman looks fine in a dress, but when she puts on shorts or a bathing suit, nobody asks her why she wants to lose weight!

Mrs. K. had been a frequent partial dieter. She had learned that she could control a good part of her distribution problem if she would lose just "enough weight." But about the first thing she said was, "I'm sick and tired of rabbit food." If the PFI diet depended on it, we could go no further. Besides, she had a special problem. Her sister-in-law came to her for lunch once or twice a week, and if it were clear that hers was a diet lunch, Mrs. K. would be teased unmercifully. So I had to solve her vegetable and her lunch problem.

"Rabbit food" of course refers to the raw vegetables, typically the celery and carrots. If a diet consisted entirely of "rabbit food," I would not be surprised at anyone's objection. But on the other hand, vegetables—both raw and cooked—are both a gourmet's delight and an excellent source of essential vitamins and minerals. As you know, vegetables of many types are included in the PFI diets because they meet our nutritional and social needs, and because they serve many purposes of our dieting program.

Some of Mrs. K.'s objections to raw vegetables were really a rejection of the idea of dieting. The more we discussed this, the more insight she developed. Then, too, it turned out that by rabbit food, she meant lettuce and carrots only (she wasn't tired of celery—she *hated* it). When I told her she could have *any* raw vegetable, there was a new light in her eyes: she liked cucumbers, green peppers, and raw cauliflower.

And then I told her how the raw vegetables could be used to make her lunches for her sister-in-law seem festive rather than dietary. I suggested that if she decorated the platters with parsley and watercress, the food would look quite different: I reminded her not to underestimate the importance of color and appearance for appetite appeal. As for the lunch itself, she could try new combinations: a delightful lunch can be made from a small (3¾-ounce) can of salmon and 6 ounces of cottage cheese. Mix them together, divide in half, and use an ice-cream scoop to put them on the plates. Surround the cheese-salmon with tomato wedges, garnish with some of the less common raw vegetables, serve with Melba toast, and forget the dessert. If that did not seem a large enough meal, she could start with jellied consommé. A good meal, tasty and colorful, and just what PFI Diet C allows for lunch!

THE 3-YEAR-OLD AFTERBIRTH

Mrs. Priscilla A. came into the office complaining that she "still had her afterbirth." I explained that inasmuch as her youngest child was three years old, it was quite unlikely, but, in any event, since I was not a gynecologist, she was in the wrong office. She smiled and explained that what she meant was that after her third pregnancy, she simply couldn't take off any weight. With her first pregnancy she had gained more than she should have, and had spent a rather trying period returning to normal weight. With the second pregnancy she was very careful not to gain too much, and more than once she told me how pleased her physician was with her.

"With my third pregnancy, however," she said, "I sure went to pot. I even cried once because I knew my doctor would yell at me. It was just such a difficult time. My first child was in nursery school, my second was into everything in reach, and then when the third was born, 'God bless him,' I was too busy to do anything. And here I am fat, and ugly, and my husband makes cracks. He should know I don't like being fat, but I don't eat much. I'm too busy with the house and kids to go to the gym three times a week! Two weeks ago my sister was in town, and she looked great. Frankly, if she can do it, why can't I?"

It didn't take long to find out why. Mrs. A. was what I have termed a *stand-up eater*. She never seemed to find time to sit down to eat. Breakfast would be coffee and nibbling from one end of the kitchen to the other. And what with the laundry, the housecleaning, marketing, making sure Billy didn't put the wrong thing into his mouth, getting lunch for the children, seeing to naps, going to buy that set of andirons which had finally been marked down, getting home to make dinner . . .

I asked her how she found time to go downtown to purchase the andirons and she said she had been admiring them for almost eight months, and she had decided she would make time to get them—even if her family had dinner late. Now, obviously Mrs. A. considered dieting as important as those andirons—because she had decided to give it prime consideration.

When we went over her food intake and added up the amount she ate as she walked about the house, it was tremendous! She purchased cookies for her children, but *she* was eating most of them.

And so I explained one of my prime rules to Mrs. A. She was, under no circumstances, ever to eat unless she was *sitting* at a table. Then, too, because she was in the habit of cleaning off her children's plates while taking them to the sink, a *second rule* was that she could have not even one-half of a bite of her children's leftovers: the food they didn't eat was either to be saved for them, or thrown out! It was true she didn't eat much at her own meals, but she certainly partook of everybody else's—including forkfuls of baby's well-buttered mashed potatoes.

The diet I prescribed for her had the standard breakfast. It took no extra time to prepare, for she could make it while she got the children's meal. Lunch appeared to be a problem, but I explained that she could eat with the children—and that if in the middle of the meal she didn't jump up to refill one child's milk glass, nobody would report her to the Society for the Prevention of Cruelty to Children. And so, lunch, dinner, and between-meal snacks could be followed as per her diet plan.

She did quite well on the diet, but not as well as I would have liked. Almost every weekly diet record that she brought in revealed a few mistakes: small ones—but too often repeated. In spite of her fairly good results, I was, therefore, concerned. Whenever I faced her with her errors, she admitted them readily. She seemed almost to enjoy being admonished. At times her entrance greeting to me was "I've been a bad girl." Her attitude seemed to be that confession would give her absolution. And after all, she could console herself that even though she wasn't perfect, she *was* losing weight.

Hers was of course the classical attitude of the child—or of the immature adult. Mommy and Daddy were always pleased with her effort, so why shouldn't I be? Besides, she knew that most parents were much more forgiving of the child who quickly, and without being asked, confessed to misdeeds. I am sure that this is why, when she was "bad," she referred to herself as a "girl." This type of expression is more immature than cute, and does not befit a mother of three! Occasionally, she would make an excuse to break an appointment and would come in the following week instead. This was, she explained, because she had had a bad week and since she didn't want to disappoint me, she had figured on making it up the next week.

Gradually she learned that admonition wasn't much fun, and secondly that I would not take the role of her parent. There would be no "A" for effort—only for achievement. I told her I had a drawer full of paper medals—but what good would they do her? I explained that there was no need to please me: I was not her judge. If she did well, I wouldn't necessarily consider her a good person, and if she did poorly, I wouldn't consider her a bad person. I was not involved in moral judgments. My job was to guide her to reduce. Confession would not help her to take off weight.

Why, you may ask, was I concerned as long as she was doing "pretty well"? Because this is the type of patient who never really learns a new eating habit and therefore is a prime candidate for regaining her weight. Back on the seesaw! As I have told you, an overweight person can rarely maintain a weight loss without learning *how* to eat.

Mrs. A. became angry with me. She had a feeling of rejection. She quit. Ten months later she returned. She had regained all but five pounds of her lost weight. Those ten months, however, had given her time to assess herself, for she returned not only apologetically, but with a new attitude. There were no more reminiscences about how pleased her obstetrician was with the way she had maintained her weight during her second pregnancy—no more appeals for my paternal approval. She now knew she had a job to do—for herself, by herself. And she understood my purpose—as guide, as instructor. No longer did she ask for absolution. I was finally dealing with a mature woman.

Mrs. A. is on her diet now and is losing weight perfectly. A complete success probably can be anticipated. Incidentally, she has refused to eat at cocktail parties, because, after all, she is not allowed to eat standing up!

THE DOUBLE PORTION EATER

Mrs. C. was about 30 pounds overweight when I first met her. She was a fascinating woman: her large variety of interests were exceeded only by the enthusiasm with which she discussed them. She had seen much of the world, involved herself actively with many aspects of it. She seemed selfless in her attitude toward life—but she had an important reason for attending to herself: she had to lose weight or jeopardize her health.

When we talked about her eating habits, she admitted she never felt completely satisfied by a meal. She would often have second portions, as well as large desserts, but at least, she said with relief, she never ate between meals.

Part of her problem could be easily solved—once I learned the symptoms. Mrs. C. was an extraordinarily rapid eater. She ate so fast that she almost swallowed without chewing. As a result, she would be finished eating before her body mechanism could signal that she had had enough—so naturally she craved a second portion or large dessert. So all I had to do was to make Mrs. C. concentrate on eating slowly.

Her other hunger had a different cause. Thanks to all of her activities, she frequently did not get to eat dinner until late; as a result, it was quite common for her to have a seven- to eight-hour wait between lunch and dinner. Few people don't get hungry during so long a period between meals.

And so I insisted that Mrs. C. have a snack in the late afternoon—to prevent an unrestrained hunger at dinner time. Simple? As I told you, details make the difference between success and failure.

One of the most significant signs of Mrs. C.'s success with her diet occurred one day just before she reached her final goal. As she was leaving the office, she stopped in front of the mirror to fix her hair. Now that she was thin, she took pride in her appearance. Even the newest clerks in my clinics notice that overweight individuals come to us somewhat unkempt in their dress, posture, and hairdo, and that it is only when they have reached the point of maintaining their desired weight that they stand straight—and proudly—are well made up, and smartly dressed. And so though many individuals think they wish to lose weight only for health purposes, there are few who do not enjoy their new appearance when they achieve it.

THE DESSERT LOVER

Evan was one of the most charming, outgoing human beings I ever met. He wore a moustache that more than half covered his face. Since his face was as full as the rest of his body, his was a formidable moustache. But he loved it—and delighted in the attention it drew.

Evan T. was a writer and world traveler. He lived well and acted as if he adored life. But there was one stumbling block to his enjoyment: he had developed very high blood pressure and he had been referred by another doctor to me.

This was not the first time Mr. T. had been told to lose weight but now he was willing to try in earnest—on his own terms. He told me he could stick to the diet I gave him on one condition: that he had something sweet at every meal.

I paid no attention to his request and concentrated on explaining his PFI diet to him: he left my office as though he would embark on it with unquestioning zeal.

He returned a week later having lost only half a pound. I went over his diet record and it was perfect—too perfect. There are few people who don't make minor mistakes the first days of a diet. I told him bluntly that I didn't believe his record. Somewhat sheepishly he said, "Doctor, I told you if I had something sweet after each meal, I would be able to diet—and I did. I stopped all between-meal eating." I inquired what sweets he had had which he did not record. His answer was astonishing: "Pie a la mode after every meal—including breakfast!"

I reviewed the diet again and re-explained the principles, particularly the fact that by following one part of the diet you are not awarded the privilege of making your own rules for another part. Furthermore, Evan T. by not recording his actual food intake was close to forgetting what he really ate.

And so if I gave him incorrect advice based on his false data, he would be the ultimate sufferer.

The next week, I had made a little more headway—but only to the extent that he left the ice cream off his pie! We had a tug of war for weeks and I was beginning to think that this was not a diet program but an endurance test. But there came the day when he walked into the office and said, quite simply, "If I'm paying you, I might as well listen to you—otherwise I shouldn't be here."

He lost weight from then on, and he was so confident of his ability to maintain his new weight that he carefully trimmed his moustache to fit his new slim self.

THE CASE OF THE PERFECT DIETER

Ethel G. was a widow in her late thirties with three boys aged 16, 14, and 12. She had been trying to lose weight since her children were infants, but had had no success with the programs she had tried. Since her husband's death a few years ago, she had resigned herself to being fat.

But now her two oldest boys had begun to press her to lose weight. She started my diet with a fierce determination. She lost weight regularly and steadily. Her graph—I always chart a graph for each patient so that both of us can follow the progress easily—was so perfect that it looked like a textbook example. She was as pleased as any woman could be. Her comment was recurrent: "Something is wrong—I get enough to eat, and yet I continue to lose weight." She kept asking me about maintenance and I kept answering her that she would have no trouble because she was developing a new eating habit.

She arrived at her new weight, and I explained the maintenance program to her in detail. But she canceled her next visit and I never saw her again.

About a year later I received a call from her family physician. He wanted to know the results of some laboratory tests that I had done on her. He told me later that she had consulted him because she had not regained an ounce during that entire year. She was concerned that she was sick since she was eating everything she liked and was still not gaining weight.

When I assured him that her tests were fine, he laughed and said "What can you do, if people don't want what they originally came for!" Mrs. G. had found it so easy to enjoy eating the new way that she couldn't believe something wasn't wrong! It seems she hadn't become used to seeing herself as a new person.

NIGHT EATING—A PROBLEM OF SEXUAL FRUSTRATION?

Mrs. Jean H. came to me with a story that can be summed up in one sentence: "I have no trouble controlling my diet during the day, but once night falls, I'm lost." Mrs. H. had two boys, three-year-old twins. Her husband was a schoolteacher. They lived in a two-bedroom garden apartment, fairly easy to tend.

Her husband faced the economic problems common to so many male teachers today, and had the added burden of contributing to the support of an ailing parent. To meet his financial requirements, he took on additional work: he coached the soccer team in the late afternoon and then taught in the adult evening school. The extra jobs provided the money needed, but made his a fourteen-hour workday, and on Saturdays he acted as a tour guide in a neighboring town.

Just what was Mrs. H.'s day? Thanks to her home duties and the children, her day was usually full but seldom stimulating. She ate her breakfast with her husband and the children, took her lunch while the twins napped, and had her dinner with the children. The boys were put to bed between 7 and 7:30, and then came the wait! A long wait! She tried to keep busy with sewing, looking for whatever child's garment had disappeared that day, reading a magazine, looking at television—and then getting dinner ready for her husband.

When Mr. H. came home dinner was ready, and she could look forward to sharing the events of the day. As they talked, she might nibble a piece of meat, join him with a cup of coffee, and a tiny piece of cake—so small that she could take another sliver. When they finished chatting, he would pick up the paper, while she cleared the table, did the few dishes, and wrapped the leftovers. But all too often, she returned to find her husband, obviously exhausted, sound asleep in the chair with the paper in his lap. She could do only one thing: awaken him gently so he could get ready for bed. And by the time she had brushed her teeth, he was in bed asleep.

Summary: Endure an unstimulating day, await one's husband eagerly, speak to him for an hour at the most, and then find him asleep. Consequence: an insufficient social life and an inadequate sexual relationship. Much desire, and no fulfillment, and yet how could she get angry with him? He was working for her and the children; after all, he didn't like fourteen-hour workdays either. The trouble was not with him but with their situation. Result: frustration.

What did she do about it? Went to the refrigerator for some leftover meat. Or tried television, but found the old comedies no longer funny. Went back for a piece of fruit. Decided she might as well finish off the small piece of cheese also. Went back to bed. Either couldn't sleep at all—or slept restlessly, and awakened after an hour. Had a bowl of corn flakes and half a piece of bread with peanut butter. And so back to bed.

Incidentally, on vacations or on Sundays, eating was never a problem! She knew too that if she visited her next door neighbors for an hour or so in the early evening, the edge would come off her tension, but she felt that she could not depend on her neighbors and encroach on their privacy.

The real problem was non-dietary. With the help of an experienced family counselor, a solution was worked out whereby the husband gave up some of his evening school sessions in order to go home at a reasonable hour. In return, Mrs. H. got a job as a part-time home typist, working on manuscripts (she had been a secretary before she married). She had plenty of time for her typing while her children napped and during the evenings that her husband worked—and so could make up the financial deficit.

Once her cause for discontent was removed, Mrs. H. stopped gorging herself, learned a new eating pattern, and began to lose weight. Incidentally, when I last heard from her, she thought she might be pregnant again.

This type of night eating is not exclusively a frustration symptom of married women with double-job husbands. For example, I had been treating a very young, shy, unmarried, 19-year-old girl who, without apparent reason, would go on tremendous eating binges. All the effort she expended on dieting was negated by her binges—binges which varied from half a dozen scrambled eggs and bacon, to three boxes of cookies and a bowl of cold cereal.

These binges occurred only at night, and it took me a long time to get her to tell me why. The young lady had a strong moral sense and an almost-as-strong sexual desire. In the course of a date, she often found herself in a necking situation she enjoyed but feared, and so she would do her best to terminate the evening. She admitted she would arrive home slightly frightened and quite frustrated, kick off her shoes, and head directly for the refrigerator. After eating, she was remorseful—but the damage was done. This girl was tranquilizing tension by using food as a sex substitute! When I explained the reason for her night binges to her, she seemed to have a resurgence of self-discipline. Later the gorge pattern reappeared, but we finally developed a way for her to stop eating before she started. All she had to do was to remind herself how guilty she would feel *after* a binge before starting one!

When I found out that still another patient of mine was constantly invading the refrigerator at night, I made what I intended as a kidding suggestion: "Why don't you put a 'What am I angry about?' sign in your refrigerator and not allow yourself a night binge until you can answer it?" One day she announced to me, "I put the sign in my refrigerator. It worked fine; I stopped eating! Then one night I went to the refrigerator in a fury, saw the question, and grabbed a pencil. I scribbled the answer 'My husband'"!

No cure of problems can come without understanding. This

patient had to realize why she was overeating. Only after she realized both that she was using food as an outlet for her tension—and that overeating did not solve the problem—could she begin to give up food as a tranquilizer.

Food as a sex substitute is not as obvious in men as it is in women. This does not mean that men are not commonly night eaters too, but the reasons for their private binges may be different. Men do most of their eating *prior* to retiring, and should therefore be called evening eaters to differentiate them from the true night eaters who awaken from sleep to eat—a much more frequent symptom in women.

Evening eating is sometimes a matter of suggestion—as with an attractive television food commercial aimed at an immediate reaction—but it is most often a manifestation of boredom and loneliness.

When evaluating night eating, I have found the eating most often to be an occupation done *alone*—a solitary diversion—a way of filling lonely and/or boring hours, or unfulfilled needs. Treatment here must be directed at the cause. There is no need for pessimism, however, inasmuch as very often once the cause is established, the answers become self-evident.

Many individuals involved in the evening eating problem have given me the impression that their problem is what to do with their hands. The answer is, use them: type, write, sew, carve, whittle, knit! If, instead of grabbing for food, you grab for a set of knitting needles or a paintbrush, you will be using your hands profitably and happily. There will be less need and less chance for putting food in your hands. After all, it is not easy to eat and play the piano at the same time. If you are lazy, you may have to force yourself to take up a hand occupation, but after a while you may discover that you are involved in a delightful recreation, rather than a system of self-discipline. So if you are an evening eater, try a hobby. You need one—and you will probably surprise yourself by liking it.

But whatever you do, remember it is perfectly normal to feel somewhat hungry four hours after a meal—even in the evening. This is why an appropriate evening snack is allowed in all diets—and why raw vegetables are suggested as hunger fillers.

THE SECRET DIETER

Before I end the section on the home dieter, let me give you an important warning: don't keep your diet a secret from other members of your family. Family cooperation is essential.

I realize that if you are a "repeater," you may be embarrassed to confess to your family that you are back on a diet. But if you don't tell them, you might find yourself choosing the path of cheating in order to avoid being recognized as a dieter. So don't create a situation that could lead to cheating. Tell your family—even your children.

CHAPTER 2

Social Dilemmas

The problem of holding to a diet while enjoying a social life is a major one for most of my patients. They complain of being caught in a food trap: the dilemma which occurs when they know the diet but the hostess doesn't. Let's see how this —and other social situations—can be handled.

THE FOOD TRAP

Mrs. L. was 38 and most charming. She had been on many diets in the past with varying degrees of success and failure. Now she considered herself faced with her biggest challenge. Her husband had received a significant promotion, but along with it came a new responsibility for her: a large increase in the amount of entertaining and being entertained they would have to undergo for him. At first it seemed to her there would be a constant stream of dinner and cocktail parties to attend with her husband. And in the past, it had always been the insistent hostess who had wrecked her diets.

Mrs. L. was also upset because she noticed that most of her husband's business associates had thin wives: "Compared to me, they're downright skinny." She told me she had to lose weight for her husband's sake and for her own self-respect. She admitted she didn't want him ever to ask himself why all the women except his wife were thin. She even asked me to put her in the hospital so she wouldn't have to face the party problem.

I told her I could hospitalize her, but that as soon as she got out, we would be right back where we started. Instead I said we would pay particular attention to "partying." The first thing she had to learn was how to say "No, thank you" to her hostess, without losing a friendship. And so I took her through the various kinds of social situations, from the most formal affairs to the seemingly simple cocktail party.

I admitted that she would be faced with many affairs at which there was no choice of food and where the food offered would be a far cry from what she was allowed on her diet. Should she avoid these affairs? Emphatically no! You don't learn a new food habit by fleeing from society. No, you must learn to handle your eating problems as they occur, so that by the time you are on maintenance, you know what to do by experience. After all, dieting is not a passive experience but an active effort composed of constant awareness and fore-thought, planning and doing!

And so I discussed the specific problems she—as well as you—might have to solve.

BEEF OR LAMB IS THE MAIN COURSE. Does this really come as a surprise? Why? They are the most commonly served meats at dinner parties, and so when you are invited to one you should anticipate that either may well be served. Plan ahead. Do not use up your beef and lamb allowance for the week and then be amazed when you find yourself served one or the other at a big event. You are old enough not to fool yourself! Watch the amount of beef or lamb in the preceding six days. Be prepared!

THE PORTION SERVED IS TOO LARGE. This is the most frequent social complaint I receive. Yet the answer to it is obvious. Do you really have to be told: "Don't eat more than your allotted portion"? I assume that others do not notice whether you finish what is on your plate. You think they do only be-cause of your own self-consciousness. Unless you spill a glass of red wine on the tablecloth, people spend more time looking at your face than anywhere else. As to that wine, if someone is pouring you more, use the universal sign language for no more: put your hand over the glass. If encouraged by the pourer, just shake your head and go back to talking to the person next to you, *but keep your hand on the glass!*

If you are really trapped by a persistent hostess who asks why you are not eating more, simply tell her that you took much too much to start and then apologize for not being able to finish her excellent food. Let her come to your rescue. She will: she will not only forgive you but will welcome the compliment. Or tell her that you have just recovered from an intestinal virus infection, and so you must still eat carefully, but you didn't want to miss her party. In other words, be cute, be clever, be funny, spread the food around the plate, but don't eat more than you are allowed.

Dinner at the boss's home offers you almost your only exception to the rule. If you feel that by refusing food you will offend your hostess and thereby the boss, think about the job and eat the food. But be honest, not easy with yourself: try just to substitute a smile for an extra bite. Similarly, if you are dining with the rich grandaunt who has willed you her money, you might decide to forget the diet. But I would prefer that if you think money that important, you try eating it!

A FORBIDDEN FOOD IS PART OF THE MEAL. This is the most sinister food trap. But there are solutions even for this stiuation. If the forbidden food is purely an accessory, simply do not eat it. Give it to your skinny neighbor if necessary. Skinny people always know how not to eat something without being embarrassed. But if the food item is an essential part of the meal—for example, if the main course is ham (not allowed on any PFI diet plan)—*take no more than half of it, pull in your belt, and think how well your diet is going.* If your self-discipline still gives you trouble, just stare at the food and imagine a dirty bug is on it. Not a pleasant thought, but it may help you to smile and starve. Fortunately, this type of food trap is rare on social occasions: your diet is based on foods commonly served.

HORS D'OEUVRES COME WITH COCKTAIL PARTIES. The problem

here is that, out of habit, people tend to pick up little hors d'oeuvres tidbits without realizing what they are doing. As I have said before, you must be conscious of *everything* you eat. You must know at all times what you are eating. If there are no raw celery sticks or carrots available, decline the hors d'oeuvres passed to you by saying you just had one: this is the time and place for the little white lies. Or try a delaying action and say you will have one later.

If you follow the Never Eat Standing Up rule at cocktail parties, you will discover that most unconscious nibbling will eliminate itself almost automatically!

And so, as I told Mrs. L., whatever the social situation, there is *never* an adequate excuse to go off your diet. All you have to do is ask yourself, "*Must* I eat it?"

If necessary, excuse yourself, go to a mirror, and look yourself straight in the eye when you give the answer. By then the host or hostess will be speaking to someone else and you can quietly murmur to yourself, "Thank you, no."

THE ALCOHOL ISSUE

I am well aware that one of the major problems of coping with social affairs is that of restricting drinking. As a matter of fact, what amazes me is not how much people drink but how little they are aware of their alcohol consumption. My patients will declare in all sincerity that alcohol does not figure in their diet, that they only take one now and then when they go out.

To determine the actual amount they drink, I ask the following series of questions:

1) Do you ever drink at lunch? How many times each week? How many drinks on each occasion?
2) What about in the afternoon (especially weekends and holidays)?
3) How many drinks do you have after leaving the office?
4) How many before dinner? With dinner (this includes beer and wine)?
5) How many after dinner? Any nightcaps?
6) And how many at parties?

And so I ask my patients to add up for themselves the amount of liquor they have in terms of times per week and drinks per time to see whether they don't drink more than they may have thought they did. Certainly most men do!

The number of different social situations involving the use of alcoholic beverages is countless. There is the college student exploring (perhaps secretly) the world of beer at a beer party. The gourmet whose meal is incomplete without wine during and brandy after. The single girl on a date who may find herself in a cocktail lounge, at a big party, or in a restaurant where an unusual wine is the specialty. The businessman who, when he goes out to lunch with a colleague, feels he has to have a drink to join his friend. The golfer who is part of a steady foursome which has always enjoyed the camaraderie of the 19th hole. The woman who enjoys a cocktail with her husband before dinner and who sometimes has an extra one by herself while waiting for him. Or the "vacationing" wife who loves a drink at lunch. The man or woman who seems to spend a good part of any leisure time at cocktail bars. The suburbanite who is mowing his lawn and is offered a glass of beer by his neighbor. Or the commuter who meets his neighbor on a rush-hour train and suggests that they try the club car for seats.

What do you do if you want to lose weight and yet do not want to give up alcohol? There are two basic methods of handling the problem. Which one you choose depends on your personal social requirements:

1) If your social (and business) life is on a regular schedule, at least in terms of alcohol requirements, restrict yourself to a maximum of one drink *per day* if your diet plan allows seven drinks per week or one *every other day* if you are allowed three drinks per week. Check page 117 where your allowance is explained. If for any reason you do not require a drink on a particular day, do not have it, *and do not make up for it by having an extra drink the next day*. If you miss having a drink, consider it as profit. One drink should meet most social and/or business needs.

2) If your social and/or business needs are irregular, re-strict yourself in terms of total drinks *per week* (three or seven depending on your diet). You may have all drinks at one sitting, or spread them out through the week. If, for example, you are dating, save your alcohol allowance for the dating days and have drinks as the social demands become evident, but never exceed your total weekly allowance. If you don't have a date that week—no drinks! And remember, from a health point of view, one drink a day while on a 1200-calorie diet means that 10 per cent of your calories are from alcohol! If you have to take someone out for lunch, save your alcohol for those occasions: but remember, the fewer drinks per lunch, the clearer the thinking.

In other words, if your alcohol social requirements are ir-regular and somewhat unpredictable, you can have a drink before, during, and after dinner, or instead have none that meal—as long as you do not exceed the weekly *total*. And re-member to figure into your weekly quota the big party coming up: save some of your liquor allowance for the occasion.

But supposing the party is unexpected? What do you do when you have already had your quota for the week? Have a glass of club soda (not sweet soda). You can ask the waiter or bartender to add a dash of bitters, and then the club soda will be colored like an alcoholic beverage. And "water on the rocks" isn't as silly as it sounds: in a small glass it looks like gin on the rocks. Remind yourself, too, that the bartender or waiter doesn't care if you drink. Besides, by now "Thank you, no" should be an important part of your diet. But if your host or hostess is truly insistent, you can always say that tomorrow you are going to the doctor for some tests and you are not allowed to drink. This is never challenged!

Finally, remember: *every drink you don't drink is profit.*

AN ALCOHOLIC TRAP. There is a different phase of alcohol's relationship to dieting that can best be illustrated if I tell you about another patient of mine. When Bill B. came in the first time, he was both arrogant and hostile. He interrupted my standard questions early, with proper apologies of course, to ask if he could make a telephone call. When I got him back to the matter of giving me information about his weight— What had he weighed as a child? Was he overweight in his teens? On entrance and on discharge from the Army? On marriage? Ten years ago? Five years ago? What was the most he ever weighed? The least? His present weight? What would he like to weigh?—he answered as though the whole issue bored him and finally he interjected: "You know, Doctor, I . . ."

I interrupted him. "Yes, I know. You want to know why you should try my diet. After all, you've lost and regained your weight a hundred times. You've been to spas, health farms, other doctors, and probably even to a hypnotist, and here I sit, not even going to offer you a pill! So let me ask you the question you were going to ask of me: Why *are* you here?"

He was taken aback by my bluntness. "Well, obviously I should lose weight, but frankly if my wife and mother (my mother's a doctor, incidentally) didn't nag me, I wouldn't be here. Let's face it, Doctor, I've made a success of my life and I thoroughly enjoy eating. So I live a few years less! I don't want a miserable diet. No one is going to make a prisoner of me!"

I told him I knew my diets were tough and so I didn't intend giving him one.

He looked at me with amazement. "But that's what I came here for! What do you mean—you won't give me a diet?"

"It's pretty obvious that eating is your most important pleasure—except possibly that of demonstrating your authority —and I will not have it said that I took anyone's greatest pleasure away."

"What do you mean 'greatest pleasure'? I've got a lot of pleasures. I don't live to eat."

At this point my secretary announced there was a call from his office for him. His response was forceful and immediate.

"Tell them I'll call when I'm done and not to disturb me. O.K., Doc, what do I eat?"

I was now dealing with an eager, cooperative patient. He

even began to enjoy the questions: Was he a fussy eater? A plate cleaner? A sneaky eater? How did he react to his wife's nagging? (He yelled back and went to the refrigerator!) Was he deprived of food in his childhood because of economic deprivation? How much alcohol did he drink?

The answer to the last question proved the most revealing. He could drink most of his friends under the table—while he entertained them with his guitar: it seems he had a large repertoire of popular songs. In addition, he would have a few drinks at a business lunch; an occasional sip from the small bar he kept in his office for when he was on edge; one or two (or was it three or four?) martinis before dinner. He didn't like wine, but he enjoyed brandy after dinner—and a few beers after golf or at a ball game. He told me proudly he could drink any amount, but added that when he drank heavily he wanted a "lot of food—especially steak." "But," he quickly added, "I go on the wagon now and then and don't touch a drop. Still, Doc, you know what I said before, I don't want to be a prisoner."

Of course, the problem here was obvious. His excessive alcoholic intake resulted not only in an enormous excess of calories, but also provoked him to gorge himself. I decided that this patient could diet *only* if he gave up alcohol entirely. It is my policy with patients who are used to extremely high intakes of alcohol not to allow them any at all while they are on the diet: it is too difficult for them to limit themselves to just a few drinks per week.

Bill was forced to abstain to the point of not even looking at a salad made with wine vinegar! He followed his diet perfectly, and lost weight according to schedule. He was proud of saying "I told you I don't need liquor. When I make up my mind to do something, *I do it!*" So far, I had no cause for complaints, but after a while his business travels began to interfere with his weekly visits. I was afraid of losing close contact with him and insisted that if he had to miss an appointment, he call me no matter how far away he was at the time. This worked out well, but one week he didn't call at the appointed time. Two days later he phoned to explain that he had met an old buddy, and before he knew it they were having an evening on the town.

Bill's visits became erratic; his phone calls equally so. His weight remained stationary for a while and then began to climb. When I tried to discuss his drinking, he countered by asking trivial questions such as why couldn't he have a large glass rather than a small glass of tomato juice before lunch. One day his secretary phoned my secretary to say he would not be in.

Of course, this man was an alcoholic. His earlier arrogance, the show of authority, were all cover-ups for his insecurity. He was a man who was destroying himself with alcohol instead of trying to cure himself with more appropriate guidance. Bill B. could never lose weight permanently until he controlled his alcohol habit.

The alcoholic must have special attention, because a difficult medical problem is often present. Some overweight alcoholics attempt to continue their drinking while they cut their food intake drastically. This is often an invitation to cirrhosis of the liver.

Fortunately, *most* alcohol problems in dieting are of a benign and social character, and as such are easily controlled.

THE VACATION TRAP

So you are going on a vacation—American Plan. American Plan of course means that the price of your hotel or resort accommodations includes meals: lots of them . . . all big . . . all rich . . . second portions easily available . . . especially desserts. . . . And all you pay extra for are the drinks! Trapped! Trapped between something you already paid for and enjoy and your diet. What are the choices?

Choice #1. Forget the diet. Enjoy yourself; you only live once. Start the diet when you return: it won't be the first time you quit and started over. Besides, maybe by the time you get back someone will have discovered a new magic way to lose weight without dieting. But if losing weight is that unimportant to you, why have you read this far in the book?

Choice #2. *Make believe* you are on a diet. Tell yourself you were so good up to now, you deserve a break. Keep on giving yourself medals: by the time the vacation is over, there should be a lot of fat to pin them on. Remember, you don't hurt anyone when you fool yourself—except yourself, of course.

Choice #3. Don't go on vacation. Be a martyr—if that will give you enjoyment.

Choice #4. Don't go to an American Plan resort. This is the first serious suggestion I have made here, but it is still a matter of choice. You may decide there is some merit in avoiding this type of resort. You may find a place with the same kind of facilities on the European Plan (where you pick and pay for your own meals). Since you are eating less, it might possibly be cheaper for you this way. Incidentally, some resorts offer both plans.

Choice #5. Go to the resort, enjoy it, *and diet!* How? By starting with the right attitude. Learn to enjoy the many delights of vacationing without making eating the highlight. Obviously, if your vacation is primarily a gastronomic tour, you can't be on any weight reduction program. But if you keep food in perspective, you can enjoy your food, enjoy your vacation, keep losing weight, and in addition leave the sodium bicarbonate at home. And when your new acquaintances discuss their resolve at breakfast time not to stuff themselves at dinner any more, you will be able to smile—knowingly.

The PFI diets contain foods and choices that should present no difficulty in resorts. The work part of dieting at resorts is to be precise, to tell your waiter how you want your food prepared, and not to succumb to his offers of more! Resorts wish to please you: they know that if they are to get you back next year, they have to make you happy. They *will* honor your requests, but you must ask. Once the waitress, whose livelihood depends on tips, understands that you really mean business, she will usually go out of her way to help.

Besides, if the portions are too large, *must* you eat them?

Dieting is your responsibility. Vacations are fun. But as there is no vacation from health, there is no vacation from dieting— that is, of course, if you really want to lose weight.

CRUISES. The cruise situation is identical to that of the American Plan resort, except that you will have a choice of early or late sittings. Usually, you have the same sitting for each meal, so the meal spacing should be even throughout the day.

ROAD TRIPS. Automobile trips may present the additional problems of unequally spaced mealtimes, and meals where the choices are very limited. So, though the same general rules apply as for resorts, you will have to take some additional precautions.

1) Watch the clock and map at the same time. Look early for a place to stop. Have your meal when you are just beginning to become hungry, rather than so late that your hunger becomes excessive. Excessive hunger makes you so irritable that you lose your resolve and may overeat. Just as a hungry driver is an irritable driver, an overstuffed driver is a sleepy one: neither is safe behind the wheel.

2) Pick an eating place in which you are reasonably sure of having choices. Don't stop at the very first diner you see. And if you don't find what you want on the menu, ask for it. All they can do is say no, but they just might have it—or be able to suggest something you hadn't noticed on the menu. And as for diners, they can all boil eggs, put "hard" cheese on a slice of bread, and serve black coffee. A little ingenuity with your ordering goes a long way.

RAILROAD DINING CARS AND AIRPLANES. If you cannot get anything appropriate, and find yourself in a real food trap, there is a rule: choose the least fatty food; take fish, poultry, or veal in preference to lamb, beef, or pork, and *then use half portions of your normal allowance*. And don't forget that you can endure being a little hungry once in a while.

FISHING TRIPS. *A fish diet* (no butter, of course) is just what the doctor ordered! And if you run the risk of "the fish were on the other side of the lake today," put a can of salmon (and a can opener) in your pack. You can still tell the folks at home you had fish for lunch!

THE FOREIGN TRIP. Foreign eating presents a two-sided problem: the pleasure of new and unusual foods and the problem of how to fit them into your diet. First, do not give up the opportunity to try new foods, but choose the least fatty ones, and reduce portions if necessary. In general, few foreign countries offer portions of the same large size that the United States does.

But watch the cola drinks, especially after the long sightseeing walks! Why not prepare for thirst by taking along some of the concentrated tablets which when put in water make a non-caloric carbonated beverage. They are sold as summer drinks (especially for children) in many supermarkets. Since they are packaged in aluminum foil, they are light and easily transportable.

A GENERAL RULE. *If you intend going on a vacation within four weeks of starting your diet, don't start the diet! Wait until your return. You need at least four weeks of appetite training to handle vacation eating problems.*

THE DATING PROBLEM

Penny R. was a Southerner who had come to New York to visit her older sister. Penny enjoyed the city so much that she took a job in a New York insurance company in order to stay. She liked her work and her new apartment, but felt that her social life was the cause of her weight problem.

The trouble was that Penny never knew far enough ahead of time what a date would consist of: a dinner, an after-dinner party, a movie-and-hamburger evening, or a ride out to the suburbs for a stop at a country inn. And on top of that, she was quite unfamiliar with many of the foreign restaurants and their unusual foods.

I told Penny that the first thing she had to do was to get up five minutes earlier to have a decent breakfast instead of waiting for the coffee break (at which she had been having coffee with cream and sugar and a large piece of Danish pastry). The night before, she could pour her orange juice, make a hard-boiled egg and put it in the refrigerator, and set up the coffee so that it would be ready when she was finished dressing.

Fortunately, the insurance company had a cafeteria with a good dietician in charge of the menu. So five days a week Penny had no trouble getting an open sandwich and a green salad. She had to supply her own dietetic dressing, but she found some fellow-dieters to share the dressing with her. She could have a glass of buttermilk with her lunch, and, if she were still hungry, a cup of black coffee. Saturdays were usually shopping days, and she would have a cottage cheese salad, without fruit—available anywhere women shop. Sundays she visited her sister and had her big dinner at noon.

For evenings, I gave Penny strict rules. Never any alcoholic drinks unless she was on a date: not even if she was out with a few of the girls unless it was an *extremely* important occasion. And never any beef or lamb as the main course unless she had a dinner date—in order to make sure she didn't exceed her weekly allotment. If she found herself confronted with rich food in a foreign restaurant, she could resort to the half-portion food trap rule.

When she started on the diet, Penny found it most difficult to conquer the problem of the late evening snack. Her custom had been either to have some scrambled eggs or a sandwich, but I told her this was a habit she would have to give up. She learned to substitute half a grapefruit or a piece of melon and a cup of black coffee. Occasionally she would have a scoop of ice cream from her allotment. If she invited a date in for a snack, she could make him eggs, while she settled for a glass of skim milk.

And so Penny found that dating was no stumbling block to dieting. Incidentally, she got married a few years ago and maintained her weight well. She gained 16–18 pounds during a pregnancy, but lost it almost immediately after the baby's birth. I haven't seen her for a while now, but I'm quite confident that she is thin.

THE LOVE PROBLEM

Signe was a pretty Swedish girl, about 22 years old. She had a good job as secretary to a rather wealthy man. To her, the best thing about her job was that her boss wanted to marry her. I couldn't share her delight: he was twice her age and already married! He gave her many promises and gifts—but an equal number of excuses. And so she remained the secret friend with secret hopes. As the tensions and frustrations mounted, Signe turned to the most readily available tranquilizer: food. She ate reasonably when her boss took her out but she stuffed herself when she was alone. She told me that one Sunday (he always spent Sundays with his family) she ate six separate breakfasts, each with bacon and eggs. Another time, she ate her way through four boxes of cookies and then, still not satisfied, went out for three almond chocolate bars!

Signe got off to a hesitant start with me. She would come late to clinic, accompanied always by a new excuse. When I eliminated her excuses she complained of digestive ailments which could be relieved only by eating. Even after many, many visits her weight loss was negligible.

It was only when she told me that her boy friend hated fat women that we began to get somewhere. I called upon the assistance of a psychiatrist to show Signe that what she was really doing was getting even with her boy friend by becoming fat—and at the same time punishing herself for an illicit relationship. As she began to understand herself, she faced the fact that she wanted to end the affair. From then on, she had little difficulty with dieting.

WEDDINGS

Finally, yet by no means last in importance, are weddings. These are frequently the most joyous of eating and drinking affairs—so much so that the prime purpose of the occasion is almost overlooked! Granted, the custom of breaking bread together was developed in Biblical times as a demonstration of friendship, but certainly there is no mention of how much bread one must "break" together. The amount we eat is not the measure of the fellowship or happiness. So the next time you sit at a wedding dinner, remind yourself why you are there. If you attend only to eat, you should not be there at all! Then, for your diet's sake, follow these rules:

1) Decide that everyone who overeats belongs to the other side of the family!

2) Be willing to say, with a smile, "No, thank you."

3) If that is not enough, say, "I just had some."

4) Try the "virus infection excuse."

5) Remember the half-portion rule for all totally hopeless food traps.

6) As I said once before, think of how your skinny table-mate would be able to reject food and liquor without embarrassment.

7) Do not forget that you are the one who wants to be thinner—once and for all!

CHAPTER 3

Occupational Dilemmas

Though, obviously, many of the occupational dietary problems are the same as those encountered in social situations, there are some dilemmas which are particularly relevant to working hours—those which my patients call job interference.

THE UNUSUAL WORK SHIFT

Some people do not work the standard 9 to 5 shift; there are many whose days begin at midday or at night. And those such as policemen who are on revolving shifts have to keep readjusting their sleeping and working times.

The thing to remember is that even if you have a job at night and sleep during the day, you are probably awake just as many hours as the day worker. And so, on the diet, you must still have three meals. No matter when you arise, your first meal is breakfast: breakfast at 6 P.M. is perfectly normal for some people. Your second and third meals are your lunch and dinner—in either order. Therefore, the rules for the night worker differ only in what time he eats—the meal spacing is the same.

THE 25-HOUR DAY

Cathy M. was young and very busy! She worked as a secretary, 9 to 5, Monday through Friday. She went to evening school five nights a week and did school field work on

173

Saturdays. What with time for transportation, she had about twenty minutes for her dinner.

She had been married for a year to a young architect who appeared to be equally busy. Except for Saturday and Sunday evenings, they usually did not see each other until about 10 P.M.—when Cathy's husband had dinner. By that time, they would both be in a state of near exhaustion. It was true that one night per week, Cathy's classes ended somewhat earlier, but there were plenty of chores to fill those extra hours: sewing, marketing, going to the dentist—or buying a birthday present. But Cathy's job was important for their finances, and she was determined not to give up her studies. And so she had tried to make the best of her arduous schedule.

Though you would think that Cathy's problem would be that of too little weight, she was heavy—just because of the fact that she seemed always to be eating on the run. Her meals consisted of a bite on the way to the office (coffee cake, juice, and coffee), tea and cookies at the office, a rushed sandwich lunch, tea and cookies again in the afternoon, a rushed sandwich dinner, and a "sort of second dinner" with her husband.

When she came to me, she was as determined to lose weight as she was to accomplish the rest of her goals. So I started her on a diet program and everything went beautifully until the third or fourth week when she complained of severe fatigue: she was in tears as she explained that she simply couldn't afford to be tired—she had too much to do.

I explained to Cathy that physiological fatigue was not an unusual occurrence. The human body has an innumerable amount of safety controls, among which is an attempt to maintain the status quo—in this case, weight. One of the ways of maintaining weight is by expending less energy. And so the feeling of fatigue can be interpreted as the body's cry to lie down, sit instead of walk, walk instead of run—in other words, to use fewer calories. It is my experience that fatigue of this type is brief, easily overcome within a week or so.

But there are psychological reasons for fatigue, too. Among them is the fact that tiredness can be a method of resisting dieting, a search for a way out of a difficult job. It is easy to say to yourself, "If it makes me feel bad, what's the point of continuing?"

I wasn't sure that I had convinced Cathy, but she returned a week later, announced that she felt wonderful, and admitted that she had given our discussion a lot of thought. She felt that her fatigue was psychological, and now that she had faced the situation, she felt fine and wanted to lose all her excess weight.

Nevertheless, it was obvious that her work and school schedule was making it unusually difficult for her to follow the diet patterns so important for success. I suggested one simple maneuver which worked extremely well: special attention to her evening snack. Since she had one hour for lunch, we planned her main meal for that time—but without dessert. Then, in the twenty minutes available before class, sometime around 5:30 P.M., she could have her supper—a light meal which would carry her through school, so that when she made her quick dash for class she was no longer starved.

When she came home from school, so that she could share a mealtime with her husband, I allotted her a snack containing more calories than I usually allow, because she had missed both her midday dessert and her afternoon fruit. Some of the night snacks we devised were:

1 oz. of canned salmon mixed with 2 oz. of cottage cheese
A green salad
1 glass of skim milk

½ oz. of hard cheese on 1 Rye Krisp
1 piece of fruit
1 glass of skim milk

3 oz. cottage cheese with ½ small cantaloupe
1 glass of skim milk

A chicken sandwich on 1 slice of thin bread
1 glass of skim milk

She could now enjoy her mealtime with her husband. Henceforth, her schedule provided no obstacles. Note again, though, that these somewhat large evening snacks are reserved for those who have their main meal at the noon hour and *do not* take either the usually allowed afternoon fruit or the main meal dessert.

By the way, when Cathy came in originally, she weighed 170 and said she wanted to weigh 140 pounds. When she got down to 143 pounds, she then said 140 might still be too high. We stopped at 131 pounds! She phoned three years later to tell me she now maintains a weight between 129 and 132 pounds.

THE DAILY LUNCH

A few years ago I received in the mail two tickets to a hit show with the following note:

> Dear Dr. Glenn:
> Ever since you have been treating P_____ T_____, we have been losing weight. You see, we have lunch with him often, and we have discovered his lunches are not only good but helpful in a non-dietary way: we no longer feel sleepy in the early afternoon. So, though we don't know you, we have decreed ourselves long-distance patients of yours and send you these tickets in appreciation. Many thanks.
> Sincerely,
> L_____ F_____
> and
> G_____ W_____

This was the nicest kind of surprise: a most flattering letter and a wonderful present—from strangers.

As to the story behind it. Perry T. was a vice-president of a television station. He was used to a big lunch with his colleagues. I showed Mr. T. how he could have a lunch that started with an appetizer, included meat, bread, salad, dessert (sometimes ice cream), and beverage—all within the PFI concept.

My only problem with Mr. T. was that it was hard to convince him that just a little more could hurt. I explained that a little more means something different to everyone. It was essential to the diet that portions be precise. And so I went over the details of how to determine portion size without carrying a scale in your pocket. I even suggested that he cut off any excess portion and have it removed from the table before he started to eat. This is an easy way to control the temptation to have another bite. After all, the temptation goes if the extra bite isn't there!

Mr. T. lost 45 pounds and has kept it off now for four years. He is a bit of a show-off and has most fun when people see him eat ice cream for dessert and still not regain his weight.

THE VARIED LUNCH

James P. was sure he could never succeed on a diet, because of his lunch problem. But Mrs. P. kept nagging him: "You're getting too fat. I don't want you to have a heart attack." When the blunt approach didn't work, she would be subtle or cute. And finally, in self-defense, Mr. P. came to me.

As he explained it, he was sure his wife could handle his breakfast and dinner requirements—might even join him, since she was not so thin herself. But his lunches ranged from a quiet bite in the office, to the expansive (and expensive) meals bought him by manufacturers who sold to his firm. Then there were the times he went out with some of his fellow employees. And once a week he had to accompany his employer on an inspection trip: the employer, a rather eccentric man, made a practice of bringing his lunch to eat in the chauffeur-driven car, and he expected Mr. P. to do the same.

So how did James P. keep to a strict diet and yet make allowances for all these contingencies?

THE QUIET BITE IN THE OFFICE. Sometimes he had a sliced chicken sandwich on white toast with lettuce and tomato (but no butter or mayonnaise), fresh fruit cup, and a cup of coffee ordered from a luncheonette. Once in a while, he asked his secretary to go down to the grocery store around the corner to pick up some cottage cheese, a tomato, and a banana for him. With the cheese and tomato, he had Melba toast: his secretary had a drawerful of packages of it because she always requested it with the hot soup which she ordered for herself from the luncheonette. Mr. P. would share the banana with his secretary.

THE EXPENSE-ACCOUNT LUNCH. Since he was not the host, it was not his prime concern to make the right impression, but at a fine restaurant or club, he did not want to order a sandwich luncheon: after all, he *did* enjoy good food. He would usually start with a vodka on the rocks (he preferred vodka and tonic, but he knew bars do not usually serve dietetic quinine tonic). The drink was of course calculated from his weekly allowance. If he wanted a first course, he frequently ordered clear consommé. He told me that once he had tried shrimp as a first course with a correspondingly smaller portion of meat for the main course, but he had not felt satisfied with the size of the meat portion, and so had never done that again.

At times, fish was his choice for the main course. But once when he asked that it be broiled without butter, the waiter questioned whether it wouldn't be dry. Mr. P. replied tactfully that he knew how expert the restaurant's chef was: the fish turned out perfectly. When he did have fish, he like bread with it, and so he had only one of his two allotted portions of cooked vegetables and one slice of bread. He ordered a green salad with a slice of lemon and, if available, some oregano so that he could sprinkle the herb on top. Dessert would be melon and black coffee.

LUNCH WITH FRIENDS. No problem here: he had the option of making it the light or the heavy meal of the day—and could adjust his menu accordingly.

THE ONCE-A-WEEK CAR LUNCH. This turned out to be easy. He would take a Swiss cheese sandwich with mustard, lettuce and tomato, some raw celery sticks as a first course, and an apple for dessert. (The employer's chauffeur supplied the coffee.) Once Mr. P. tried a half sandwich (Swiss cheese) and a hard-boiled egg, but he said the egg was too messy to eat in the car.

DINNER ENTERTAINMENT

Arthur D. was an aggressive businessman. It was important to him that he make good, and early. His middle initial was I., and I decided that it probably stood for impatient. He was so impatient he quit college after 2½ or 3 years and went to work. He was in the real-estate business with a national concern which raised large amounts of money to purchase major properties. Mr. D. had a double job. Half the time, he was taking prospective investors to dinner at which it was his function to be nice to them. The other half, he was being induced to purchase properties, and so he was the one being treated nicely. And, as he said, "The niceness was always over a dining table where food and liquor were in seemingly unlimited abundance."

His weight had been creeping up but he hadn't paid much attention to it until one day at lunch when an investor had started a story with "We fat people . . ."

And thus I met Arthur who wanted to know how soon I could get the weight off him. The answer was of course only as soon as his body could burn off the fat through a diet which would allow him to stay healthy and still learn good eating habits.

Mr. D. was worried enough about his appearance to stick to the diet I gave him—and worried enough about disguising the fact that he was dieting to prepare some stock openings for entertainment situations.

1) When he was doing the entertaining, he would stress that he wanted his dining partner to eat and drink well. Mr. D. would save his own liquor allowance for these situations. He would order a drink, but then say to the waiter, "Bring me a glass of water first; I'm very thirsty." His partner rarely noticed that he did most of his sipping from the water glass and so made one drink last through two of his client's.

As for food, he found that if he manipulated his guest into

ordering first, the client would not notice what Mr. D. ordered. Furthermore, he would make it a practice to start his meal with consommé, so that it would seem as though he was having a large dinner.

2) When he was the guest, if his host insisted, "You must try this restaurant's six-flavor whipped cream cake," he had an answer ready. "It sounds wonderful, but my doctor has me on one of those new anti-cholesterol diets, and since I get my blood test tomorrow I better not." Then he could quickly add, "What does your doctor think of this cholesterol business?" And if they both found enough fault with the medical profession, the food consumed would be overlooked and the necessary rapport established.

When he was being entertained while on a business trip, he had a different set of excuses: "I always have trouble adjusting to different water while traveling. So I had better eat lightly." Or "I love to fly, but the speed of traveling seems to take away my appetite."

Mr. D. made his search for excuses a personal challenge—and enjoyed it. For he discovered that he was bright enough to figure a way out of most situations. Of course, when he was caught in a food trap, he used the emergency rule of eating only a half portion of an incorrect food item.

But one of the most important things he had to learn and did was that when he went to conventions, he could never, never make up for a night's festivity by skipping breakfast the next day. The diet breakfast *starts* each day's diet!

Part IV

The Stages of Dieting

Now that you have seen how others have handled special dieting problems, let's get back to yours. By now, you have started your PFI program—hopefully with the necessary enthusiasm and determination.

EARLY PROBLEMS: THE FIRST WEEKS

LIQUIDS. Probably during the first week on the diet, you found yourself so preoccupied with putting something in your mouth that you had a fairly high fluid intake. As the diet progresses, however, you will gradually consume less liquids than you did even before you began.

Note that you are allowed *reasonably* unlimited amounts of certain liquids: think in terms of your own body. Obviously, if you are restricted in your use of salt, do not drink club soda unless it is the sodium-free dietetic type, and stay away from bouillon. If your digestive system cannot handle coffee too well, don't drink too much of it. And if coffee keeps you awake at night, try a decaffeinated variety—or switch to tea (it has as much caffeine as coffee does, but for some people is a better before-bed drink).

CORRECTING MISTAKES. I realize that since the diet is new to you, you will make mistakes. Remember not to try to make up for yesterday's mistake by eating less than you should today. Your diet does not allow much leeway, so if you take less than the diet calls for, you may become excessively hungry, and thereby find yourself weakened in resolve and ready for more cheating—a vicious circle. If you go wrong, then, the only way to correct your mistake is to get back on your diet— *and this time stay there.*

GASTRIC COMPLAINTS. *Constipation* can be a real problem, but it is almost always a temporary one. There are simple reasons for its occurrence:

1) The decreased fat in the diet may result in decreased bowel lubrication or in decreased bile flow.
2) The decrease in food intake usually results in a smaller bowel movement.
3) After the first week of dieting, there is often a decrease in the fluid intake.

You need not be concerned unless you feel uncomfortable. If you do, drink more water and eat more raw vegetables. Have your fruits raw rather than as juice or cooked. If a laxative seems necessary, consult your physician. But do not use prune juice or prunes: too many calories per portion.

If you suffer from *gas*, try cutting down on your raw fruits and vegetables for a few days. It will usually help. If it doesn't, see your physician.

AN END TO INDIGESTION. You will be pleased to know that for most people, a PFI diet causes an end to the gastric disturbance which so often plagues the overeater. Even those patients who have never admitted to indigestion tell me, after they have been on the diet for a few weeks: "You know, Doctor, I just realized that I no longer take anything for upset stomach or heartburn at night!"

THE FIRST DANGER PERIOD: THE THIRD WEEK

You know the expression that everything happens in threes. Well, it seems to be true of dieting. At least to the extent that there are three distinct danger periods: the third, the sixth, and the ninth week of dieting.

The first week, despite its exigencies, usually ends with a pleasant surprise: most people lose *double* and some even *triple* the amount specified in their charts. The late Dr. Norman Jolliffe gave two explanations for this. He said that the fat lost early in a diet is the so-called "soft" fat which contains a high percentage of water. Furthermore, many people have a hidden supply of excess water (occult edema) in all their tissues, a supply which diminishes greatly at the beginning of a diet. I would add that since at the start of a diet you decrease significantly your total amount of food, you decrease at the same time the total amount of salt you ingest. And since the body's salt is responsible for the amount of fluid retained, the less salt, the less the fluid. This is, I believe why urination increases at the beginning of a diet, even to the point of waking you up at night. Then, too, as I said before, many dieters drink more water than usual in the first week. If there is a low salt content to this water, it may actually remove additional salt from the body (medically, this is known as "diuresis from hypotonic solutions") and consequently further fluid loss. (This water loss shows on the scale as additional weight loss, but is not fat loss.)

The excess water loss often continues during the second week, and so it is fairly common for the scales to reflect a weight loss 1½ times that predicted for you for the second week. By the way, I have noticed that the amount and duration of the more than predicted weight loss appears to be related to how overweight the person is. The extremely overweight individual can lose four times the predicted amount the first week, and may continue with excess loss for many weeks. The slightly overweight individual may lose very little extra, if any, and then only for a few days. All persons, however, should achieve at least the predicted weekly weight loss.

The third week, however, often brings disappointment: the dieter may lose *less than* the predicted weekly weight loss, may possibly lose nothing, and sometimes may even gain a fraction.

A chart showing the typical weight loss of a patient on the diet for the first ten weeks is shown below:

CHART OF WEIGHT LOSS

Predicted weekly weight loss = 2 pounds per week

	Weight	Weekly loss	Total loss	Predicted total loss
Start	154			
End of				
1st Week	149½	4½	4½	2
2nd Week	146¾	2¾	7¼	4
3rd Week	146	¾	8	6
4th Week	144½	1½	9½	8
5th Week	142½	2	11½	10
6th Week	142	½	12	12
7th Week	139¼	2¾	14¾	14
8th Week	137¼	2	16¾	16
9th Week	135½	1¾	18½	18
10th Week	133¾	1¾	20¼	20

The inadequate weight loss in the third week is explained by one of two factors, and often by a combination of both. First, there is a tendency of dieters who do well at the beginning of a diet, particularly if they are losing *ahead* of the predicted weekly weight loss, to pat themselves on the back a little bit, become overconfident and decide that they have the diet licked—and so can go off it a little. One of the reasons, then, is the dieter's worst offense, *cheating*. The other reason is that there is usually a readjustment of body water balance: as the eating pattern begins to achieve some regularity, the balance shifts and some water is now retained. If salt intake has been increased, the water retention will become even more accentuated.

The water balance situation in the early weeks of the diet may be described in terms of a pendulum: an excessive swing in the first week to the side of dehydration and a return swing the third week to less water elimination. Unfortunately, pendulums never seem to stop exactly in the middle.

And so comes the end of the dangerous third week when people tend to become discouraged because of their apparently diminished weight loss. It is all too common for a patient to say: "What's the point of dieting if I can't lose weight?" This is why I call the third week the quitting week.

Remember, as long as you are on your diet, you are burning fat and losing fat weight no matter what the scale shows. The water balance situation may simply prevent it from being obvious. Go back to your weekly weight chart, and *if you have followed your diet 100 per cent,* your *total* weight loss for the three weeks will be no less than the predicted total weight loss for the same period. If it is not, re-examine your diet to find out where you are not following it precisely. (Did you have five, instead of four, dinner portions of beef one week—just because you used up your quota before the Saturday night party? Remember, dieting requires thinking, planning, and doing!) By the end of the fourth week, if you are dieting correctly, your weight loss will probably equal the predicted amount, and then you will know that you can be successful.

The Second Danger Period: The Sixth Week

This is another stage at which the dieter develops a feeling of overconfidence, but now it is usually combined with a certain degree of boredom. Since you are the only one who can determine how important it is for you to lose weight, you will have to decide whether it is worth the boredom. For most people, it is. So this is the time to put the side blinders on. Stop rationalizing and stay with it. *This is the hard drive.* You probably are not at the right weight as yet, so don't quit!

Part of your problem will be to avoid listening to those well-meaning, or apparently well-meaning, self-appointed advisers—the people who tell you that you have lost enough weight already:

1) Your spouse. Sometimes a husband will tell his wife that if she loses too much she will look like a boy. And some women feel that a thin husband doesn't look virile. There is no one-sentence answer to those who have preconceived notions of proper body size in relation to sex, except that weight is no test of virility or femininity. If it is obvious that a body-image concept may be a problem, then discuss it with your family physician.

And there is another factor: a certain degree of competitiveness between husband and wife. I have had a few cases in which a wife had nagged her husband to lose weight, and when he finally did she had seemed subconsciously to resent the fact. It was almost as though the loss of weight had changed their relationship. Here, again, a physician's help is needed.

2) Parents and in-laws. Most frequently, from this group comes those who are the most encouraging (and/or nagging) to see you start to lose weight, and yet are the first to say you have lost enough. In general, I advise most of my patients simply to disregard the suggestion. After all, this book is written for adults, and you can act as an adult with your parents also!

3) *Fat* friends and associates. Thin people rarely tell you to stop losing weight; fat people often do. Why? What's your guess? Mine is jealousy!

If you want to fool these friends, just wear tight clothes. People judge your appearance more by the way your clothes fit than by anything else except your eyes and the shape of your face.

If you have rings under your eyes, people will say you don't look well because you have lost weight, but the odds are that the real reason is that you are tired. Get a good night's sleep.

Many people will comment that your face is thinner. The reason for this is that the loss of even part of an inch of fat in the face is quickly noticed, while few of us can see even a loss of two or three inches at the waistline. But people will get used to your new facial appearance—so don't worry about it. And I assure you it is not one-tenth as bad as envious people might lead you to believe. Just realize that if the rest of you was too fat to start with, your face was probably also too fat. And this book is not meant for people who want to keep fat faces.

THE NINTH-WEEK DANGER

At this time, the danger is discouragement. You may have made a few mistakes along the way, so that your batting average is only 80 per cent. Since it is now over two months since you started dieting, you again face the tendency to weaken your resolve, to think that maybe your present weight is good enough. It is a natural psychological trap. You won't be the first to experience it, but most people work their way out. So continue on your diet and stay on it. You are probably not done yet. Since with the end of the tenth week, you will reach your first re-evaluation time (to see how far you still have to go), give an *extra* push to reach that period. And if you find yourself having real trouble with your diet, do the following:

> Omit all beef and lamb for one full week.
> Substitute chicken, fish, shellfish, or veal.

Dieting can be likened to taking an automobile trip from New York to Chicago. You start off in New York, with much determination; in spite of traffic lights, road jams, street construction, and giant building cranes that block traffic, you make your way through the tunnel or bridge and onto the Turnpike. The way now is open, and progress is constant. You are getting nearer and nearer to the goal. A short stop for gasoline throws the mileage-time record off a bit, but it doesn't matter: you are soon back on the road again. But it is still a long way to Chicago, and the ride is becoming somewhat monotonous. Perhaps it is time to stop and rest a bit? Or perhaps you should take a short side trip and continue on later? Maybe even change the itinerary completely and not go to Chicago? Of course, if it is important for you to reach Chicago, you will keep to the route, put up with the monotony, and drive until you reach your goal.

The end stage of dieting, like the long drive, *is* monotonous. But the goal is up to you. In my experience, the patient who decides to stop short of his goal is usually the one who will not maintain his weight loss.

Let me tell you of one patient who had a long road to travel. Donald B. had about 80 pounds to lose when I saw him for the first time. He said he was sick and tired of being overweight. It was getting more and more difficult for him to tie his shoes; his indigestion was keeping him up at night; and the last straw was when his boss said, "Don, the kids in the shipping room have a running bet as to whether Tony, the ex-wrestler, is strong enough to pick you up if you fall. So watch out for banana peels!"

Mr. B. was so determined to lose that he was a perfect dieter. He lost 28 pounds the first ten weeks and 25 the next ten weeks. The following five weeks he lost 10 pounds and the next five weeks 2 pounds. But then the excuses began pouring in—always convincing but more and more trivial, and often accompanied by a sheepish grin. His sheepish grin began to give him away. Mr. B. had so thoroughly enjoyed the congratulations of everyone about him that he had already pinned his medal of achievement to his breast pocket. Now it was fun being kidded about his weight—because of all he had lost.

This was the time to make him face things squarely. I offered him my drawer full of paper medals but told him he shouldn't forget that it was only in grammar school that one gets "A" for effort. And I reminded him he was still 15 pounds short of his goal. I asked what his reaction would be if his son, then a high-school senior, announced he was quitting school with only three months to go. Mr. B.'s response was instantaneous: "I'd murder him," he said. "With three months to go, it would be idiotic." And so I got across the point that his quitting with seven weeks to go was equally idiotic.

I suggested to Mr. B. the trick of buying a new suit which was a little too tight, so that he would feel fat again and redevelop a new drive. Mr. B. understood. He lost the remaining weight. He has kept it off now for about four years.

Time for Evaluation

Every ten weeks of your diet, you must stop for a moment, and re-evaluate your progress until you reach your final goal.

At the end of your first ten-week period, then, take a good look at yourself. Are you as thin as you would like to be or have you more weight to lose? Go back to your diet selection chart and by using your new weight as a guide, find out if you should change to a new PFI diet and *how much* weight you should lose each week. Make a notation of this on your weekly chart. If you are scheduled for a diet change, look up and read the new diet. Read it and reread until you have learned it. Compare it with your previous one and try to understand the changes. And to make sure you are dieting correctly, check the earlier material on how your diet works.

But of course what you want to know is just how much you should weigh. Theoretically, your ideal weight is that at which you not only look your best but feel best and are healthiest.

There are two rough guides that most people can use to determine their best weight. I claim no scientific accuracy for them, but they are so frequently correct that I must mention them. For most married women, the best weight is what they were when they got married. For many men, their best weight is the lowest they weighed in the service.

Now for the scientific methods of measuring optimum

weight. The *best* single weight guide—and the one used by most physicians—is the chart of height-weight standards based on the 1959 Build and Blood Pressure Study. It lists, as desirable, weights which are in general not only lower than average but also lower than those considered desirable 20 years ago. As I helped to point out in an article in the *Journal of the American Medical Association* a few years ago, the significance of these new height-weight standards is great: *they give the weight level at which most people have the longest life expectancy.*

I have had many patients say, after I have told them their probable ideal weight: "I have never been that low, at least not since I was a child. I couldn't adjust to *that* weight." My answer is a question: "Just because you have never been rich, does that mean you couldn't adjust to becoming wealthy?"

In the Appendix are separate charts for men and for women in which I list, according to frame and height, what I consider your *maximum* desirable weight, based on the latest standard height-weight charts. And because it is difficult for many people to judge their body frame, I have included in the Appendix a description of how to determine whether your frame is small, average, or large.

If, after you have studied the charts, you still feel the weight indicated is wrong for you, let your physician decide. By using methods now available, he can measure your skin folds with special calipers to determine the actual amount of fat present.

Incidentally, the new height-weight charts no longer include age as a consideration: the older adult is not "entitled" to weigh more than the younger one. The problem for older people who have been overweight a long time is that their skin may have become so stretched that it will sag noticeably when the overweight is reduced—thereby producing a haggard appearance. This is all the more reason why you should lose weight when you are younger, *before* your skin has stretched to the point where the elastic fibers have torn and will not pull back again.

Overweight individuals almost always look younger when

they lose weight. In fact, after losing much weight a patient of mine who was in her early twenties once was asked to prove her age before she was served a drink in a cocktail lounge. A nice bonus for good dieting!

Part V

CHAPTER 1

Exercise, Massage, Automation, and Steam Baths

I have saved until now any discussion of exercise, massage, massage machines, and steam baths as ways of losing weight, because it is not until you are well on your way to achieving your correct weight through the PFI diet that you should consider any of these—even the best—as body aids.

EXERCISE

Let me tell you first the experience of a doctor I treated. Dr. Matthew R. was such a well-known surgeon that he was busy from early morning to well into the evening, and very often went back to the hospital in the middle of the night for emergency surgery. There were times when it seemed to him that he worked eight days out of seven.

He had done well on his diet, and had only a few more pounds to lose when July first came. July was family month for Dr. R. He turned his practice over to a colleague, and took his wife and four children off to the coast of Maine where they had a house in a rugged area. To Dr. R. vacation was as intensive a period as work: swimming, hiking, water-skiing, volleyball and long bicycle trips were all part of the routine. The result was exercise all day! Dr. R. watched his diet, but had no scale to determine his progress.

When July ended and he came back to my office, his reaction was: "Your scale is wrong! I must have lost more than 1⅜ pounds in four-and-a-half weeks!" An angrier man would be difficult to find. "I used more muscles than I did playing college soccer!" he exclaimed.

We reviewed his vacation diet. He had been eating berries constantly—a low-calorie food—but he covered them with heavy sour cream. Heavy sour cream has the same calorie count as heavy sweet cream! When I pointed out a few more errors, he realized that exercise will not compensate for a broken diet.

I know that physical fitness of Americans—particularly of the youth—has become of nationwide concern. But unfortunately, too many people interpret physical fitness purely as muscle fitness, without taking into account the other factors needed for physical health. Nevertheless, such a discussion is not germane to my book: you want to know what role exercise plays in adult weight control.

First, there is no question that the perpetual sitter will lose weight at a lower rate than the pacer. After all, it is a simple fact that every calorie "walked off" is one less calorie worth of stored fat. So if we multiply these "walked-off" calories, we *can* walk off weight. The problem really is how much can we walk off? A measurable amount? Well, a walk of one mile will result in the loss of approximately 1/70 of a pound or about ¼ of an ounce. No, not very much and not measurable on any scales we generally use. If we quadrupled this by walking four miles, we would lose 1 ounce—again not very much. If we settled for two miles a day (walking one mile a day in the morning and one in the evening) the result would be a half-ounce loss each day. Also not much and not really measurable—but if these walks were taken 365 days a year (including rainy days!) they *would* result in a weight loss of 10 to 12 pounds per year.

The difficulty is that to lose a half-pound or more by most kinds of exercise requires so much effort that the result is often quite taxing, unless, of course, the body is adjusted to it. Then there is the problem that exercise is often associated with additional thirst and hunger. Who doesn't want a drink or two or three after a game of golf? (And overweight people tend to like high-caloric drinks.) And who doesn't have a large appetite after two or three sets of tennis? Why do you suppose so many bowling alleys now have bars and coffee shops?

Of course, if you weigh yourself just before, and again just after exercise, you may well find a distinct weight loss. Why? Simply because it is quite easy to lose 2 pounds from perspiration alone. In warm weather football players will sometimes lose 8 pounds in a few hours. Since the body requires water balance, the water the athlete drinks after the game is retained, and so his next day's weight is just about the same as it was prior to the game.

Weight loss is dependent not only upon the type of activity but on your ability. For example, the professional golfer swings with less effort, has to swing fewer times, and walks a straighter line than most golfers and so burns fewer calories. But the nonprofessional athlete cannot always make the time to do a sufficient amount of exercise regularly.

Many charts have been designed to show how many calories are expended during various physical endeavors. Here is a chart which demonstrates the point a little differently. I have converted calories to their equivalent in food products—some of them the food you would eat right after the activity.

EXERCISE CHART

Sewing for 1 hour	=	1 small ginger snap
Dishwashing by hand (main meal, family of 4)	=	1 slice of bread
Painting walls in the house for 3 hours *without a stop*	=	One 12-oz. can of beer and 4 oatmeal cookies
Walking 1 mile in the morning and 1 mile in the afternoon	=	2 pats of butter
Sitting on the beach for 3 hours	=	½ Coca-Cola
Swimming for ½ hour	=	1 ice-cream soda
Bicycling for 1 hour	=	2 doughnuts
Most types of active exercises (per hour)	=	1 Tom Collins and 3 potato chips

So though I am not against exercise, I do not advocate it as a method of weight reduction *except in amounts unlikely to provide excessive thirst or appetite demands.* (If the dieter would ignore his appetite demands, or treat his thirst with plain water, we would have no problem, but I am dealing with human nature and the eating habits of the overweight!) Therefore, if you want to exercise, think about forms which fit the formula. After all, it would be foolish not to realize that the 10 to 12 pounds that can be lost yearly by two one-mile walks daily is real weight loss. And this type of exercise should not affect thirst or appetite. So do some more walking.

Exercise does have a different—but definite—role in the weight reduction program: to *tone* the muscles (make them firmer). Muscle toning can be a significant aid in getting a trim figure, but you should not start exercise for this purpose until you are *within 5 pounds* of your final goal. Until then concentrate on your diet. When you are ready for muscle toning, consult the many good books on exercise regimes. But don't rush into extensive exercises: build up gradually. And remember that for women, modern interpretative dance classes are one of the best methods. Above all, evaluate your own ability: for example, though a hard swimmer uses many muscles, if you are a floater you are letting water buoyancy work for you.

MASSAGE

Massage is a form of passive exercise, and since not even active exercise helps much with weight reduction, it must be obvious how little muscle punching, kneading, and rubbing can do for you. It may make you feel great, but it offers no help in weight loss, except possibly for the masseur or masseuse.

SPOT REDUCING. The reduction of only one specific area of the body is constantly sought after but rarely achieved. *There is no known satisfactory medical method to spot-reduce fat.* Though there are drugs that can selectively put fat in certain areas of the body—and I don't advocate them—there are none that can significantly remove fat from a specific area. And, though muscles can be toned by exercise, the duration of this tightening depends on the frequency and constancy of the exercise. Even the professional ball player gets flabby soon after he stops playing ball.

Though we cannot truly spot-reduce, there are ways to hide fat:

1) Maintain good muscle tone. Keeping muscles tight will not lessen fat but will give the impression that there is less fat.
2) Pay attention to clothes and tailoring. The use of proper foundation garments, vertical stripes, careful choice of skirt styles—and the many tricks of good tailoring and dressmaking are important.
3) Watch your posture. Look at some of the "before and after" ads in the magazines, and note the posture in the "after" pictures. Good posture helps.

But, above all, remember one thing: trying to spot-reduce by massage is ridiculous. Fat is living tissue; it is enclosed in microscopic cells that can no more be pushed away than can muscle cells or bone cells. Visualize massage moving fat from the left buttock to the right buttock. Silly, isn't it?

AUTOMATION: MACHINE REDUCING

I have sometimes thought that the problem of the overweight individual can be said to have started and supposedly ended with machinery. The start was the invention of machines that not only took away the need for use of your own arms and legs, but also allowed more time for indulging in eating. And the solution of the problem was another kind of machine—one that jiggled the fat up and down or left to right, or was strapped to your feet and moved your legs as if you were riding a bicycle. While the latter was working, you could either sit or lie, and if the constant motion didn't bother you, you could even eat another box of candy while the machine was doing the work for you.

A variety of machines are offered to the patient who wishes

to lose weight. Their advertisements often consist of large but vague promises—promises left open to the reader's interpretation. For example, these advertisements will often quote inches lost, but will not say for how long. They may add, in small print, that if you wish to lose weight, a diet may also be helpful! (The exclamation point is mine.) And, of course, they mention how easy it is for you, how little *you* must do. The inference is: "Plug it in—the machine will do the work for you!"

The most common types of machines in use today are:

1) Those which apply rollers to various parts of the body.
2) Belt vibrators.
3) Electrically operated muscle vibrators which stimulate the muscles to contract.
4) Machines that move your feet or arms electrically and thereby imitate the movements of bicycle riding or rowing.

Most of these machines are equivalent to an "electric massage"—in other words, to another kind of passive exercise. Those machines which contract the muscles electrically will tighten the muscles—but not for long. For example, flex one arm and see how tight you can make your biceps. Now release it. What has happened to all that tightness?

Nevertheless, if you enjoy having your fat jiggled, your feet rotated, the muscles alternately contracted and relaxed, by all means plug the electric cord into the outlet (or get someone else to bend over to plug it in—it's easier that way), and go to it. And if you want to obtain a machine inexpensively, try the used-products section of the Sunday newspaper classified ads; you will undoubtedly find one offered for sale by a *still fat* person.

You may prefer to go to a salon for your machine exercise. Then you can enjoy the operators' chatter, luxuriate in lotions and oils, straighten your posture, be measured all over, and accept all compliments graciously. Don't forget to grunt and groan a little to give the impression that you are working very hard, and don't lose the opportunity to share your problems and miseries with your fellow sufferers. And at the end, take a vigorous shower: it will give you a sense of accomplishment.

But don't expect to lose weight in the process.

Steam Baths

Steam baths are a form of delight to some and torture to others. The only significant weight loss they produce is from perspiration, but if after you have emerged you drink a glass of water, the water will be retained by the body and the weight lost from perspiration all regained.

Summary of Non-Dietary Aids

I do not want it said that I take all the fun out of life, so:

If you like golf, play it.
If you enjoy massage, have one—manual or electric.
If you like the steamy feeling, take a steam bath.
If you want to lose weight, *diet!*

Measurement Difficulties

BODY CHANGES

There are some patients, perfectly willing to follow the PFI diets without detouring for non-dietary aids, who are perplexed by optical or psychological illusions in the process. Some are sure they have lost weight without losing inches. Others that the inches have diminished without weight loss. Neither of these statements is true, but I can tell you why at times it would seem as if both of them are.

When you are *very* overweight, there will appear to be little measurement loss in the early weeks of dieting. There are two reasons for this:

1) Most overweight people are wearing tight, barely fitting clothes when they start on a diet. Thus the initial weight loss merely allows them to fit into these clothes, even though the weight loss may be equivalent to a full size.

2) It is not easy to observe an inch or two loss in waist circumference if you were 250 pounds at the start of your diet. If you weighed 130, however, and then lost two inches in waist circumference, it certainly would be difficult *not* to notice the change.

The more weight you lose, the thinner you become, and the more obvious is the measurement loss. But you must be patient about measurement changes. They will appear to occur with increasing frequency toward the end of your diet. Thus, when you lose your last 5 pounds, your measurements will change more noticeably than they did with the first 5-pound loss.

Yet at times the reverse is true: when patients are astonished by the fact that they have lost in measurements but not in actual weight. This usually means that there has been a body water retention. In women, it is most often observed during the pre-menstrual period.

Illusions to the contrary, measurements are reduced all over —but the greatest loss is seen in those areas where the fat accumulation was the largest.

UNDESIRABLE RESULTS. An important point is often raised by women whose excess fat is primarily below the waist. It seems to such a dieter that in order to achieve her desired fat loss below the waist, she must lose too much from her bust and face. Sooner or later, she will have to decide whether or not to stop reducing further in order to avoid unwanted bust and face fat loss. But before she makes this decision, she should be told about *maintenance* weight distribution.

During weight maintenance, my patients have often shown what seems to be a redistribution of fat. Those areas that showed the largest fat loss in the early stages of dieting now seem to fill out somewhat. At the same time, there is a continued fat loss in those places where little loss occurred at the beginning of the diet. I do not have a scientific explanation for this, but it is a clinical observation that I have made many times!

PLASTIC SURGERY. If you were extremely heavy at the start of the diet, and have been thinking about plastic surgery for the removal of excess skin and fat tissue, do not have it done until you have assured yourself that your weight loss is permanent. This requires 6 to 24 months. Otherwise, you will risk stretching operation scars.

CLOTHING CHANGES

Sometimes the first change noticeable to women is the

seeming lengthening of skirts—the result of loss of fat over the hips. Men will usually notice first a change in their waistlines —as shown by the belt notch needed. Other men will think their shirt sleeves have lengthened: the answer is the loss of shoulder fat. Shoe and collar sizes will change, and upon occasion even the size of your gloves.

This of course brings up the question of tailoring, alterations, and new clothes buying. And so we have now reached the most expensive part of dieting. Unfortunately, even if you have a closet full of old, smaller sizes, you may find that by the time these old clothes fit, the styles have changed.

I would like to make the following suggestions:

1) In the beginning of your weight loss, avoid expense by doing only the most essential alterations.

2) Since your diet will usually continue beyond one season, don't buy any clothes for the season in which you start.

3) If you want much backslapping and kudos, then wear your largest clothes; everyone will think you have lost even more weight than you have. Large shirt collars are very effective for men!

4) I do not recommend that you take the third suggestion seriously. Instead, get rid of your old clothes as soon as they do not fit. Unless you are handy with a sewing machine, have a minimum of alteration done, because it will often be inadequate by the time the clothes are returned from the tailor or dressmaker.

5) When you *do* buy clothes, buy them a little tight. By the time cuff or hem-length alterations are completed, they will fit better. And if they are still somewhat tight, they will serve as inspiration for you to lose more!

6) Avoid any *major* clothes buying until your maintenance measurements appear to have stabilized. Measurements often vary during the early weeks of maintenance.

7) Admire your final appearance and take pride in the compliments of your tailor or dressmaker. This is one of the satisfactions of your achievement.

Are you tired of vertical stripes? Try the plaids—they will look good now!

As I said, clothes and tailoring are the most expensive parts of weight reduction, but I think you will find the result is worth the expense.

By the way, make sure your rings do not fall off: you may have to have them made smaller—or buy a guard ring.

Part VI

CHAPTER 1

Maintenance

So you think you have reached the right weight and are ready for maintenance? First of all, make sure you didn't stop 5 to 10 pounds short of your goal. One of the most essential things my patients have to learn is: don't start maintenance because "you can't lose any more." You *can* lose as much as you need to lose. Maintenance starts with your correct weight, not when you become too lazy to continue dieting. The weight seesaw is not fun—as you know!

The real test of the effectiveness of any diet is of course the permanence of results *after* dieting. I tell all of my patients that if they satisfy two conditions during the diet, I can show them how they can *eat anything they want and still not regain weight!* These two conditions are:

1) That they follow my diet *precisely.*
2) That they achieve a weight that we both agree is best for them.

Does this sound impossible? Well, it isn't. But lest I be accused of quackery, look carefully at what I said. First, I said *show them:* I cannot maintain their weight for them. As I have said from the beginning, I can show you how to lose weight, but you, not I, are the one who must do the actual reducing. Also, I did not say that my patients could eat *anything* once they reached the maintenance stage but rather *anything they want.* There is a big difference in these two statements. You see, precise dieting carried out without any cheating until a perfect weight is achieved will result in most people *wanting* to eat differently from their pre-diet habits. This is the result of the appetite retraining from constant, persistent dieting—a process of learning based on repetition. And it is the natural development of the new eating habits learned from the PFI system.

Not too long ago, a patient in the terminal stages of her diet kept threatening me at every visit: "The very day you say I can stop dieting, I am going to go directly to the nearest soda fountain and eat an ice-cream sundae." She had been dreaming of it for months and could describe it perfectly: strawberry ice cream, topped with whipped cream and a cherry. When the day came that she reached her right weight, she headed triumphantly for the drugstore. The next time I saw her, she was somewhat shamefaced as she told me what had happened. "I sat at the counter and looked in the mirror behind it. There was my new thin face. I realized how stupid I was being. I didn't want the sundae. I guess I just wanted the freedom to have it. I settled for a cup of black coffee. Now I know what you mean when you said I can eat everything *I want.* I enjoy my new weight too much to give it up for a sundae. I doubt that I will ever crave such things again."

THE MAGIC MARK

When you reach your correct number of pounds, the number immediately above it is called "the magic mark." If, for example, your ideal weight is 120, then your "magic mark" would be 121. Actually, you should continue dieting until you are about 3 pounds under the magic mark. Thus, if your mark is 121, you should get down to 118, 2 pounds below your ideal weight of 120. This is to give you a leeway area (118 to 120), since you cannot be expected to maintain a weight precise to the ounce every day.

As long as you are below the magic mark, continue eating anything you wish. Of course, if you eat six eggs, bacon, and a side dish of pancakes for breakfast; two corned beef sandwiches and potato salad for lunch; meat, fried potatoes, and pie a la mode for dinner—all in one day—you certainly won't keep your weight down! I'm not really worried though: by the time you achieve your ideal weight, you won't want to eat this way. But that still doesn't mean that any of these items are now forbidden to you. You can have them, but in moderation. As I told you, you diet with your head—by thinking. You maintain the same way—with your head.

On maintenance, weigh yourself daily! Most people weigh themselves in the morning before getting dressed, but you can choose any time, so long as it is the same time each day, and you have on the same amount of clothing (or lack of clothing). If you ever reach, or go above the magic mark, then *immediately* return to your diet—and follow it strictly for a full twenty-four hours. You should be able to take off your surplus weight within the twenty-four hours. But if you are still above the magic mark the next day, stay rigidly on the weight reduction diet. Don't put it off—don't wait until after the weekend: *this is the biggest cause of failure.* When you are once again below the magic mark, you may go back to eating what you want.

In the beginning you may find yourself two days below the mark and one day above, as if you were on a pendulum, but as you learn to avoid excesses, you will still be able to eat what you want and keep the pendulum swings both smaller and less frequent. Remember, however, that even though you certainly do not have to diet all your life, you will have to be very conscious of your eating habits—and your daily weight—for many years to come.

Most users of the PFI diet system have found that if they keep to a fairly constant diet-type breakfast and lunch, they have considerable leeway at dinner, where there is usually the biggest food demand. But if you ever get into trouble—remember the basics of PFI:

Watch the *P*ortion sizes.
Watch the *F*requency of foods such as beef and lamb.
Watch which *I*tems you choose.

Conclusion

Conclusion

Conclusion

Many years ago, someone used a weight reduction method that appeared to be ideal: it allowed you to eat anything and still lose weight, and all you had to do was take one single capsule at the start. It appeared to work perfectly, but in time its users became anemic, developed digestive complaints, complained of fatigue, and then discovered they had to go through a very unpleasant medical procedure: they had to be dewormed!

The original capsule had contained the head of a tapeworm! The tapeworm grew and grew. It utilized the food eaten for its own purposes instead of letting the dieter's body absorb it. The tapeworm became healthier and healthier; the individual developed poorer and poorer health and finally had to be hospitalized.

Fortunately, there are governmental methods of stopping this type of treatment: a cure by disease! But though parasitic infestations—a major cause of disease—cannot be used to prevent overweight, something must be done to put an end to this problem.

For overweight is a serious health problem. I would estimate that close to 40,000,000 adults in the United States alone are overweight. And they are overweight to an extent that not only shortens life expectancy but increases both the early development of disease and the amount of disease to which a person is prone. And, as we have seen throughout this book, overweight is also a cause of frustration in daily activities and thus takes its toll in our emotions.

Overweight occurs in affluent, food-abundant societies—and among affluent individuals in food-poor countries. It is truly everywhere. It is found among the rich and the poor, the active and the inactive, the tall and the short, the smart and the dumb, the famous and the unknown, the ambitious and the lazy.

And yet the overweight person can diet successfully as long as the motivation is not simply a desire to be thinner, but a willingness to learn how to eat differently combined with a willingness to follow what has been learned. After all, anyone who has bought this book doesn't need to be told why to lose weight—just how.

The methods, experiences, and ideas related in this book are those that appeared to me to be the most significant among those patients who succeeded in the PFI diet. They were the ones who were willing to accept the fact that though good dieting is hard work, it is the *only* way for most people to lose weight permanently. A good way of dieting (there is no such thing as only *one* good way) has been described here. If the law of averages holds true, by the time this book is published, a new method of weight reduction will have been devised. Obviously I cannot evaluate it ahead of time. But you can do your own evaluation by asking yourself the following questions:

1) Will it allow me to lose weight and stay healthy?

2) Will it allow me to meet my three most important dietary needs: my home, my social, and my occupational food needs?

3) Will it allow me to learn new eating habits so that I will be able to maintain my weight in the future?

4) Has it been tried fairly and successfully by a sufficient number of persons?

My colleagues often kid me and call the above "the four postulates of Glenn." I probably shall still be kidded, but I insist that every dieter be able to give an affirmative answer to all four questions.

Appendix

Food-Shopping Hints for the Dieter

COST

You start by saving the money which would have been spent on cakes, butter, candy, and other forbidden foods. But that doesn't mean you shouldn't take care to get your money's worth.

First of all, watch the scales and *read the labels*. Do not be fooled by packages that appear large or use the term "large size." Go by the weight: after all, you need to know package weights for your portion control. It is usually cheaper to buy the largest package or can that you are able to store, but if tiny, individually-packaged items aid you in your portion control, it might be well worth the extra few pennies to buy the single portion sizes (the individual serving of cereal, the 3¾-ounce fish can, etc.).

And for both dieting and money saving, buy only as much as you and your family should eat. Don't allow for leftovers. They can be too tempting and will lose food value and flavor if kept too long.

BREADS. Check the label to make sure the bread is enriched. Remember that special "diet" breads are often so termed only because they are cut in thinner slices: do not spend extra money just because the word "diet" is written on the package.

Bread is almost always cheaper than rolls, and so you will be saving money by avoiding another forbidden food.

MILK AND CHEESE. Skimmed milk and cottage cheese are inexpensive products. Evaporated (not condensed!) skim milk is available. Yogurt is generally a more expensive form of partially skimmed milk. And to save money in the hard cheeses, stay with the domestic rather than the imported types.

FRUITS AND VEGETABLES. Shop early in the morning. You get a better selection, and therefore more for your money. If orange and grapefruit juice are out of season and quite expensive, use tomato juice for your morning citrus fruit. Depending on the season, canned fruits and vegetables may be less expensive than the fresh, but if canned remember they must be water-packed. Simple water-packed fruits are often less expensive than "dietetic fruits," and you can add your own artificial sweetener as desired.

ANIMAL PROTEIN (MEAT, POULTRY, FISH, AND EGGS). As you know, poultry and fish are often cheaper than beef or lamb and so it will cost you less to meet the preferred protein requirements. Then, too, there are other savings to be made in this category. Frozen fish fillets are often less expensive than fresh fish. Canned pink salmon is cheaper than canned red salmon; canned water-packed dark tuna is cheaper than canned water-packed white tuna; solid pack is more expensive than grated or flaked canned fish. As to eggs, buy the cheapest color your market sells. Color of the egg shell does not affect flavor or food value.

So you see, you need not spend more money to eat less!

FOOD GRADING*

Grading is done by the U.S. Department of Agriculture for two purposes: for the consumer and for the wholesaler. Only

* For more information, write to Superintendent of Documents, U.S. Government Printing Office, Washington 25, D.C. for Home and Garden Bulletin No. 58 (Shopper's Guide to U.S. Grades for Food)—price 10¢.

consumer grading will be discussed here. Grading in general applies to the quality of food *at the time of grading*. The use of U.S. grading is strictly voluntary, and is paid for, if requested, by the food producer, processor, or handler. Graded foods usually have *U.S.* in a shield-shaped mark on the label, and, except for meats, are designated by letters: U.S. Grades A, B, or C.

Marking of meat is done with a purple vegetable juice which is *harmless* and usually disappears on cooking.

MEATS

Only an official grader of the U.S. Department of Agriculture can use the shield with the letters U.S.D.A. and the proper grade name. Meat is graded either by whole carcasses or wholesale cuts, not by small retail cuts. Individual cuts may therefore vary from the grading, in spite of marking. If meat is marked "U.S. Insp'd. & P'S'D," it means that it was inspected and certified for wholesomeness, but otherwise not graded as to type of quality. Examination for wholesomeness must be done for meat shipped in interstate commerce; meat shipped in foreign commerce; and meat to be quality graded.

BEEF. There are six grades of beef for retail use:* U.S.D.A. Prime, Choice, Good, Standard, Commercial, and Utility. All six of these will provide satisfactory, wholesome food.

Prime. This is the top quality. It is well interspaced with fat and is tender and juicy. Most of these cuts go to hotels and restaurants.
Choice. High quality, but less fat than prime beef.
Good. Less fat than choice, but fairly good quality. Less juicy but still tender.
Standard. Very little fat, but can be very tender if prepared properly.
Commercial. From older cattle, and usually less tender. Requires long slow cooking with moist heat.

---

* Two additional grades, Cutter and Canner, are rarely offered to retail tail customers as fresh beef, but are used in various sausages and other processed meat foods.

Utility. Least tender. Almost no fat. Economical for stewing and boiling.

Now you can see that the grading of meat is mostly on its fat content. In general, remember, the higher the grade, the more fat, and the worse therefore for the dieter. I must admit that an unscrupulous butcher sometimes adds pure fat to lower grade meats to make them appear juicier and of higher grade, but most local laws prohibit this.

LAMB, YEARLING MUTTON, AND MUTTON. The grades here are five: U.S.D.A. Prime (there is no prime grade for mutton), Choice, Good, Utility, and Cull.

Mutton is uncommon in the United States; 90 per cent of sheep marketed for meat are lambs. In addition to their higher content of fat, the higher grades have a smaller percentage of bone.

VEAL AND CALF. The official grades are: U.S.D.A. Prime, Choice, Good, Standard, Utility, and Cull.

Veal is usually from animals less than three months of age. Here, too, there is more fat and less bone in the higher grades. But there is not as much fat as in beef or lamb, and since it is not intermingled with the lean meat, it is therefore more easily cut off as visible fat. In general, moist heat is necessary for preparation. Calf, which is from a slightly older animal (3–8 months), also has a high proportion of lean to fat.

PORK. As you know, this is not allowed on the PFI diets in this book. To my knowledge, Federally graded pork is not available to the consumer.

POULTRY

Here too we have two marks: the inspection for wholesomeness and the inspection for grading. There are three Federal grades for ready-to-cook poultry: U.S. Grades A, B, and C. This grading is done for chicken, turkey, duck (not allowed on diet), geese (also not allowed on diet), guineas and squabs. Grading is based on shape of the bird, neatness, amount of fat under the skin (again the more fat the higher the grade), as well as bruises and discoloration.

Eggs

Many states require grading, and eggs often are labeled as graded under Federal-State supervision. *The grades and weight classes are entirely separate and unrelated to each other*: a small egg may be of low or high quality; the same is true of the larger sizes.

Eggs are graded as follows:

Top quality: Fresh Fancy Quality
U.S. Grade AA
U.S. Grade A

Lesser quality: U.S. Grade B
U.S. Grade C

Eggs of the lesser quality usually have a thin white that spreads over a wide area when broken, and also a flat yolk that breaks easily. These eggs are best used for cooking with other food ingredients.

The U.S. weight classes are:

Jumbo (30 oz. to the dozen)
Extra Large (27 oz. to the dozen)
Large (24 oz. to the dozen)
Medium (21 oz. to the dozen)
Small (18 oz. to the dozen)
Peewee (15 oz. to the dozen)

The first and last of these classes are rarely found. For your diet, *use only Large or Medium eggs*.

And remember, the color of the shell does not affect the quality of the egg!

Butter

As you know, this is not allowed on your diet, but for your general information: Butter must have the prefix "U.S.," or it has not been certified by the Federal Government, regardless of any grades written on the package. Sometimes grading is done by the state. Federally graded butter is designated as:

U.S. Grade AA (U.S. 93 score)
U.S. Grade A (U.S. 92 score)
U.S. Grade B (U.S. 90 score)

"Score" is the total number of points given a sample of butter and is based on various quality features such as body, texture, etc., but mostly on flavor.

CHEESE

Grading of cheese is less common in consumer packaged cheese.

The grades for cheddar are U.S. Grades AA, A, B, and C.

The grades for Swiss cheese are U.S. Grades A, B, C, and D.

Grading of cheese is mostly on flavor, texture, and body.

There are no U.S. grades for cottage cheese, but it may be labeled with a U.S.D.A. "Quality Approved" shield.

NONFAT DRY MILK (skim milk)

Though grades have been established, they are mostly used for commercial trading.

FRESH FRUITS AND VEGETABLES

This is a complicated classification, since there are 84 standards for 71 different produce products for the grower and wholesale shopper, and 13 standards for consumer use. U.S. No. 1 is not always the highest grade, for in some food the terms U.S. Extra Fancy and U.S. Fancy take precedence over U.S. No. 1. In general, consumer standards use alphabetical designations (A and B) rather than numbers. The size is marked next to the letter: U.S. Grade A—Small; U.S. Grade B—Medium to Large. There is no marked difference in the *nutritional value* of the first and second grades of the fruits or vegetables.

One of the big problems with grading these products is that by the time they reach the consumer they may no longer be in the same condition as they were at the time of grading.

PROCESSED FRUITS AND VEGETABLES

These products range from canned fruit cocktail and tomato juice to peanut butter and pickles. Here also there are a variety of grade labels. In general:

> Grade A—Fancy
> Grade B—Choice for fruits
> > Extra Standard for vegetables
> Grade C—Standard

Height-Weight Charts

Before you can use the following height-weight standard chart, you have to know how to determine your *frame* or your *bone size*. Because the charts are based on frame, some people cannot use them: the unusually muscular individual (such as an active professional athlete); the person with markedly different bone sizes in various parts of the body; the individual with exceptionally large chest expansion and massively broad shoulders. The charts are also not for those who have severe curvature of the spine resulting in shortened height; those who have had an amputation, or those with atrophied muscles (as may occur after poliomyelitis).

To determine your frame, I suggest two methods:

1) *Wrist size.* Look at your wrist. Is it small (we call it petite in women), average, or rather large? This is a wonderful judge of bone size in my experience.
2) *Shoe width—not length.* In most instances, foot length is a measurement that goes along with body height. *Width* of feet, however, is a fairly good measurement of bone size. Narrow feet indicate a small frame; medium width an average frame; very wide feet a large frame.
3) *Hat size.* This is a good method for men. Follow the same principle as with the other methods.

229

Even with these rules, I know it is not always easy to determine your frame. But I can tell you that most people are of *average* frame, whether or not they have a lot or very little fat on their frame. If you are still in doubt, use as your standard the frame size *smaller* than you think you might be.

Please note the heading on the following charts—for women and men. I cannot give you your exact desirable weight since this would have to be established individually for you by your physician. And so the figures given are a guide to the maximum you should weigh.

MAXIMUM WEIGHT FOR WOMEN*
WEIGHT IS WITHOUT CLOTHES**
HEIGHT IS WITHOUT SHOES

Height	Small Frame	Average Frame	Large Frame
4'8"	95	104	116
4'9"	98	107	119
4'10"	101	110	122
4'11"	104	113	125
5'0"	107	116	128
5'1"	110	119	131
5'2"	113	123	135
5'3"	116	127	139
5'4"	120	132	143
5'5"	124	136	147
5'6"	128	140	151
5'7"	132	144	155
5'8"	137	148	160
5'9"	141	152	165
5'10"	145	156	170
5'11"	149	160	175
6'0"	153	165	181

* Adapted from Metropolitan Life Insurance Co. For women between 18 and 25, subtract 1 pound for each year under 25.

** To determine weight with shoes and clothes, add 2 to 5 pounds.

MAXIMUM WEIGHT FOR MEN*
WEIGHT IS WITHOUT CLOTHES**
HEIGHT IS WITHOUT SHOES

Height	Small Frame	Average Frame	Large Frame
5'1"	116	125	137
5'2"	119	129	140
5'3"	122	132	144
5'4"	125	135	148
5'5"	129	139	152
5'6"	133	143	157
5'7"	137	148	162
5'8"	141	152	166
5'9"	146	156	170
5'10"	150	161	175
5'11"	154	166	180
6'0"	158	171	185
6'1"	163	176	190
6'2"	167	181	195
6'3"	171	186	200
6'4"	175	191	205

* Adapted from Metropolitan Life Insurance Co.
** To determine weight with shoes and clothes, add 3 to 6 pounds.

Index